D0071707

Living Time

Living Time

Faith and Facts to Transform Your Cancer Journey

BERNADINE HEALY, M.D.

BANTAM BOOKS

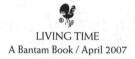

LIVING TIME
A Bantam Book / April 2007

Published by Bantam Dell
A Division of Random House, Inc.
New York, New York

Library of Congress Cataloging-in-Publication Data

Healy, Bernadine.
Living time : faith and facts to transform your cancer journey / Bernadine Healy.
p. cm.
ISBN 978-0-553-80461-4 (hardcover)
1. Cancer—Popular works. I. Title.

RC263.H394 2007
616.99'481—dc22
2007002588

Printed in the United States of America
Published simultaneously in Canada

www.bantamdell.com

10 9 8 7 6 5 4 3 2 1
BVG

To cancer patients
past, present, and future

And in loving memory of
Michele

PREFACE

THIS BOOK IS MEANT to be a gift to those who are, have been, or will be touched by cancer. It is a disease that strikes like lightning and takes us down a road that challenges our being in a universal way. But we live in a magical time in which cancer's secrets are giving way to the sharp eye of science; under its gaze, cancer treatment is also becoming more humane and personal. The cancer journey is full of turning points and crossroads, hills and valleys best navigated by an informed patient and family. You must be willing to challenge current dogma, stay engaged, have a healthy sense of humor, and above all, have faith in yourself, in what you hold dearest, and in your own tomorrow. This is my hope for you.

CONTENTS

Living
Time

PART ONE

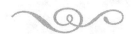

The Start of My Journey

When I dipt into the future
  far as human eye could see;
Saw the Vision of the world,
  and all the wonder that would be.

—"LOCKSLEY HALL,"
ALFRED, LORD TENNYSON

CHAPTER 1

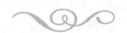

A Valentine's Day

S O THIS IS HOW I DIE.

These words ran through my mind as I lay in the emergency room of the Cleveland Clinic on Valentine's Day, 1999. It was in the wee hours of the morning, a time I remembered all too well from my medical residency years at Johns Hopkins. That's when the ER would fill up with drunks and drug addicts, knife and gunshot casualties, car accident survivors, and early morning heart attack victims. Many years had passed since then, but now I was one of them, an emergency room patient in great distress. I had just received startling information that would forever change my life.

Only a few hours earlier, my husband, Fred, and I were sitting up in bed watching the Oscar De La Hoya fight on HBO. At some point that I cannot recall, I passed out, only to awaken with the local rescue squad standing by our bed. I was confused. Why were they talking to

Fred about my ambulance ride to the hospital? Why was my husband on the phone with his good friend Al Lerner, asking him to meet us in the emergency room? I protested that this was all unnecessary, that I felt entirely well. I had an overwhelming desire to stay and comfort our terrified twelve-year-old, Marie, trembling in the shadows, and to talk to Michele, my sister, who'd rushed over to be with her. Despite these protests, I soon found myself strapped to a narrow gurney in an ambulance with flashing lights, hurtling along dark, deserted streets into midtown Cleveland.

Dr. Patrick Sweeney, the gentle, white-haired neurologist who was the attending physician that evening, met us in the ER, ready to perform the usual neurological tests for what my husband believed had been a seizure. Fred is a renowned cardiac surgeon and at the time was the director of the Cleveland Clinic, but he was pure husband that night. He listened attentively to Dr. Sweeney and acted as the best of spouses would, making sure I was comfortable, squeezing my hand, and calming my nerves with lighthearted jokes: "Hey, was this just your way of getting out of watching the prizefight?"

But very shortly we found that my blackout had not been an inconsequential seizure after all. Fred knew first because he went off to huddle with the radiologist to review the brain scans. He stood quietly by, eyes swollen, as Dr. Sweeney brought me the shocking news: the spell had resulted from a good-sized tumor growing in the left side of my brain. I asked Dr. Sweeney if it was malignant. Leaning over the rail, peering into my eyes, he said simply, "Yes."

Even though Fred and I have an uncanny ability to think the same thoughts at the same time, this was one moment when we could not bear to share those thoughts. After all, we always said we were goose and gander, mated for life; we wouldn't do well without each other. And all I could think was: *So this is how I die.* Not in a car accident or a plane crash, not felled by a heart attack in honor of my own medical specialty. It would be by my own cells, mutating and roaming inside my body—in my head, no less. I felt powerless and immobile. My own life's work with the critically ill brought me no special strength or solace; if anything, I knew too much. This cancer was insidious, already having grown to a near-fatal state in my brain without ever tipping me off. Not one hint.

Here I was in the prime of life, and fairly diligent about all the healthy habits I had preached so reverently for decades. Though a cardiologist by training, I had also earned my stripes in the war on cancer: I was then the dean of the College of Medicine and Public Health at Ohio State University, where I had been expanding the school's cancer genetics program. Years before, I had headed the Research Institute of the Cleveland Clinic Foundation, where I built its first cancer biology department. And as director of the National Institutes of Health in the early 1990s, I oversaw the National Cancer Institute and participated in its 1991 celebration of twenty years of the National Cancer Act, which brought us the war on cancer. There I also immersed myself in the massive effort to unravel the human genome, which will have its greatest payoff in the area of cancer. And in the course of my life as a hands-on physician, I had cared for and consulted with patients who had had a brain tumor. I had every reason to know the meaning of my newly diagnosed illness. It was not good.

At that long moment of discovery, looking up into the sad, drawn face of my husband, I knew that all of our medical expertise combined would not help us cope with this numbing news. No matter who we are, from whatever background, we all feel the same chill upon hearing the C word. It's a universal fact: when serious illness strikes, we are the same vulnerable souls.

And so are our families. Returning home the next day, that became all too evident. Their world, too, suddenly becomes cloudy. It was hard to explain to those on the home front what still seemed inexplicable to us. To my ninety-eight-year-old mother-in-law, Nonie, who lived with us, this was bewildering news. Her "Bernie dear" was never sick. As for my mom, cancer was the thief that had taken my dad from us twenty years before, and it was not hard to see in her pale, stoic face that she knew what might be in store. How good it was that she had moved right next door to us several years before—although the plan then was that we could look after her, not the opposite. Things also changed for my sister Michele, who was part of our family compound, too. Her protective big sister was suddenly the weaker one. My heart swelled with gratitude when she whispered in my ear that if it was needed, she was ready to offer up her bone marrow or anything else she could to get me through this. But what proved hardest for me were those lingering hugs from my two girls, twelve-year-old Marie, who had been up all night, and nineteen-year-old Bartlett, who rushed home from college. Moms are supposed to be there when you're growing up, after all, and the sinking feeling that it might not happen for them was obviously written all over my face. As I surveyed my treasured nest, I knew that this illness was not only about me. I had just managed to rock my family's universe, and it was going to be my job to keep that in mind as I navigated this journey.

I recollect this traumatic time not to torment myself or to unsettle you, but because I have come to understand that in slogging through the dark valley of cancer I experienced another dimension of life. Confronting and surviving this disease compelled me to do a mitzvah, a good deed, in the only way I know how—by writing this book. As a physician who has cared for the seriously ill and spent a lifetime immersed in almost every dimension of health and disease, I was now the vulnerable patient. Through it all I've acquired some hard-won insights that just might help others facing a similar predicament—insights that I so dearly would have valued but were not clearly evident to me at the time. And they came not because I had a unique experience that turned out better than expected, but rather because I lived an all-too-common one. Only in retrospect can I see that my illness turned out probably as it should have, but not as well as it will in the future for others who will have the means to find it sooner and extinguish it faster. The common denominator for us all, in the still early morning of this new century, is that we are witness to a mighty sea change in the life of medicine and its war on cancer.

But back to the home front. My husband got the wheels in motion. He arranged for the surgery that would be performed a few days later by Gene Barnett, his colleague and director of the Cleveland Clinic's Brain Tumor and Neuro-Oncology Center. Dr. Barnett would remove as much of the tumor as he could. With tissue in hand we would nail down precisely what variety of tumor showed up as a nasty white blotch on my scans and map out the next steps. Though he did not spell it out to me in such detail at the time, Dr. Barnett believed the tumor was what's called a glioma. A glioma is a tumor that arises in the brain's glial cells (astrocytes and oligodendrocytes), whose function is to create supporting structures for neurons, or nerve cells. Cancers are usually graded from I to IV based on how nasty they look under the microscope. He speculated mine was a grade III glioma made up of a mix of both forms of glial cells. This was one step from the summit on the glioma malignancy scale, the summit being the more common variety known as glioblastoma multiforme, or GBM. I pressed Dr. Barnett as to what his diagnosis would mean for my future. His answer was sobering: with a full course of treatment, including surgery and radiation and possibly follow-up chemotherapy, I might have one or two good years, maybe more; with surgery alone, it would be less. In either case, the outcome would be improved if he was able to remove the entire tumor. But that was the rub, and a big one. The tumor was in an unlucky location: on the left side of my brain.

Like most people, I'm "left-brained," as evidenced by my right-handedness. If I had to have a brain tumor, I knew from my basic medical training that having it on my dominant side was not the best news. The situation was even dicier because the mass sat near the brain's speech center. Speech, like handwriting, can be dominated by the left or right side of the brain, or controlled by both. (You have heard of ambidextrous people. There are also some whose

speech is "ambi.") If by some stroke of good fortune my speech center happened to be located on the right side of my brain, or present
in both brain hemispheres, the risk that removing the tumor could
damage my ability to speak would be eliminated. So, prior to surgery, I would have a special test to determine something most of us
never need to know—exactly where all my chatter was coming
from.

But figuring this out was not so easy, as I was soon to discover. It
required an invasive procedure that would delay surgery for a couple
of days. The procedure was very similar to a coronary catheterization—it was even done in a cath lab—except that the catheter was
threaded into the carotid arteries that feed the brain rather than into
the coronary arteries that feed the heart. Called the Wada test, after
the Japanese neurologist Juhn Wada, this clever study sorts out the
activities of the right and left parts of the brain by selectively putting one or the other hemisphere to sleep with a slug of short-acting
phenobarbital.

The radiologist started off with my left carotid artery. As my left
brain went to sleep, I instantly went mute. I was awake, alert, focused, and trying very hard as he asked me repeated questions. The
words lined up in my head, wanting to be released, but instead just
piled on top of one another like a nasty car wreck, at first one sentence at a time and then full paragraphs. I simply could not get them
out. I suddenly felt the frustration that I have seen in the eyes of
stroke victims who—despite the fact that they see and hear, feel and
reason—are fated to keep that all locked up inside their head. It did
not escape me that in a matter of a few days I had gone from being a
healthy person to one experiencing a cancer, the likes of a cardiac
catheterization, and the sensibility, however brief, of a major stroke.

As for me and Wada, I flunked the test, at least as I hoped it
would turn out, so much so that the radiologist saw no value in even
finishing the study of the other side. My speech center was located
near the tumor, making the operation that much more difficult for
Dr. Barnett—and yes, for me, too. One thing was now clear in my

mind: however much time I had ahead of me, I did not want to wake up from surgery unable to say thank you or communicate any other thought or feeling. My husband and I, each in our own way, relieved Dr. Barnett of any urge to be heroic with his scalpel; that is, we preferred he err on the conservative side of how much he could remove safely. As Fred put it most simply and plainly: "I want my wife back."

There was a lot to do before surgery. I had to convince Marie that the tiff we had had the night I fell ill had nothing whatsoever to do with causing my sudden visit to the ER. It turned out that I was more successful doing that than at convincing our college sophomore, Bartlett, that brain surgery wasn't such a big deal. Seyhan Soylu, Marie's godmother and a close friend to both Fred and me, dropped her work in Columbus and moved into the guest room for a week, shoring us all up with her warm and quiet strength.

I also had to put my professional life in order. I took on the task of canceling my appointments at the medical school for the next four weeks, meetings that no longer seemed so earth-shatteringly important. Those that were, I'd do by phone. "No problem; don't yet know for sure what it is; a little brain surgery and I'll be back in a few weeks." I listened to myself repeating these facts strongly and confidently, when I felt so weak and wimpy. But clear-voiced and confident was for me the way to go; wearing my fears on my sleeve only made them scarier. One of the axioms I live by is Never scare the children—including the one inside you.

With the outcome of the Wada test in hand, Dr. Barnett gave me the option of being awake during the portion of the neurosurgery in which the tumor was actually being removed. I jumped at the idea of being awake with a purpose—being a sentinel for my own speech center. By speaking aloud on the operating table, I would assure Dr. Barnett that his cutting was staying away from my speech zone. I've done a ton of public speaking in my time, but this recitation would become the most important speech of my life.

The operation began like all others, as Dr. Zeyd Ebrahim, the neuro-anesthesiologist, let me peacefully doze off while trying to count to ten. This gentle sleep was abruptly broken when he brought me back to full consciousness in the midst of the operation. My face peered out from under the large green drapes. Behind me I could hear Gene Barnett's soft voice and the ever-present sucking sounds of the OR. More important, I could speak, feel my body, and wiggle my fingers and toes, though I was clearly harnessed to the operating table, with my head immobilized by some kind of paraphernalia. I had no pain, mental or physical. Dr. Barnett had already numbed my scalp with a local anesthetic and opened up a four to five-inch window into the left side of my skull to expose the tumor. I discovered all too personally what I had learned long ago in medical school from lectures about the legendary Harvard neurosurgeon Harvey Cushing: the mind can suffer mightily, but the brain itself is incapable of feeling pain, even if tugged, cut, or singed. Cushing was famous for doing brain operations on people who were wide awake.

My brief reverie was interrupted when neurologist Hans Luders, an expert on brain geography, appeared before me in full surgical garb. How strange it was to see him there. The last time I'd spoken with him, we'd been talking about nerve cells he had been able to grow successfully in a culture. He now stood over me holding my neurosurgical homework—a literary passage I was to read again and again during the operation. This was strangely satisfying: I was part of the team, aware of what was going on, able to influence my own outcome, never entirely relinquishing whatever meager control over my fate I could muster.

Like a third grader reading aloud in front of the class, I tried to pronounce each word perfectly, though the words seemed odd. I asked Dr. Luders if this passage made a lot of sense to him, and he laughed. To me, it seemed out of context and very flowery, not at all a passage that I would have chosen for this critical moment in my life. But, hey, who was I to be choosy? Just as I was feeling comfortable about my ability to handle this strange experience, Dr. Barnett told me he was finishing up and all was well. Hans made an exit, and

Dr. Ebrahim put me back to sleep. The next awakening was to my smiling husband, daughter Bartlett, and dear friend Seyhan. Dr. Barnett had removed about half of the tumor and had plenty of tissue for further studies, including some newer genetic analyses that were just beginning to identify differences among subtypes of gliomas.

While in the hospital I had my first meeting with another member of my slowly assembling tumor team, a group that I soon affectionately called my brain trust. The pediatric neuro-oncologist Bruce Cohen, who happened to have a lot of experience with gliomas in both children and adults, came by to see me. A soft-spoken, scholarly man in his forties, he had a wise rabbinical way about him. It was easy to share my thoughts with him—my hopes about being there for Marie's last year in middle school, and for Bartlett's college graduation in two years. We talked philosophically about those joyous life events that we all share yet are so personal to each individual. I mentioned my husband's greenhouse, where amidst his many orchids he created an intensive-care unit for seedlings and newly grafted trees. I wanted to see those trees grow strong and tall in the outdoors. I had dreams of seeing my daughters find their right mates, and maybe even become parents themselves. My stepdaughter, Alison, had just had little Wyatt, and Fred and I had all sorts of plans for him. I was also fully expecting to see Nonie turn one hundred; to see Michele become a grandmother; and to see Mom, the family seamstress, make the christening gown.

Perhaps that was too much to hope for right then, but these were no idle thoughts, and Dr. Cohen knew it. I wished to remain the wife and mom my family knew, and that meant a return to my everyday professional life as well. I had just made a great effort to protect my speech center, and I was no less dedicated to the preservation of my brain. I have always been driven by brain, not brawn, and I wanted Dr. Cohen to know exactly what this meant to me.

It was too early to discuss the specifics of my subsequent course of treatment with him while the tumor was still being analyzed in the laboratory, but this preliminary conversation was critical to laying out just how I felt about what I expected from therapy. I already knew that radiating the brain was the conventional and near-universal approach; chemotherapies were deemed second string and usually ineffective. I confessed to a bias against brain radiation; it was easy on the rest of the body but invariably damaged at least some healthy brain tissue. Though the kinds of chemo that were in use or on the experimental horizon were rough on the rest of the body, they spared the brain. Dr. Cohen was sympathetic to my personal thinking on this but gently warned me that chemo alone would be seen as "malpractice" by at least some of the experts in the field.

When we received the pathology studies several days later there was some good news. My tumor was of the less common variety, called an oligodendroglioma (as opposed to the more common astrocytoma), a rather obscure tumor that was just starting to make a splash because of its unusual genetics. Dr. Cohen gave me a brief tutorial on work currently being done in Canada at the University of Toronto, where recent studies suggested that at least one subtype of this tumor, when it carried a particular genetic profile, was surprisingly responsive to therapy—including chemo. He did not want to get my hopes up, but he said Dr. Barnett was to perform genetic tests on my tumor, with results in a few weeks. If it fit a particular gene profile called a 1p-19q deletion (in which hunks of chromosomes 1 and 19 are missing), there was an increased chance that I might have an enduring response from chemotherapy and that radiation could be forestalled, if not avoided entirely.

He cautioned me again, however, that opting for chemotherapy alone was not standard care, or, in today's parlance, "evidence-based" care. Instead, what he described to me was in essence the emerging strategy now known as targeted treatment—I'll discuss that in detail later—in which therapy is tailored to match a given person's tumor genetics and to his or her personal life choices.

There were no conclusions reached that day—it was only two

days after my operation—but this meeting set the stage for many decisions that would be made in the weeks and years ahead. I fervently believe that this kind of straight and personal talk is one that cancer patients must have with their doctors early on. Though one needs the guidance and perspective of the doctors—I later met with several other doctors who had their own views and would become part of my medical team—never for a moment did Fred or I lose sight of the fact that we were the ones who would live with whatever choices were made. And that's true for every patient.

Before I left the hospital, Dr. Barnett stopped by to unwrap my head bandages. For the first time I realized I still had most of my hair. I never thought to ask about it before surgery, but there it was covering up that long incision and making me feel quite unchanged. In fact, it gave me a little jolt of confidence as I went home to face the next phase of fighting this cancer, diminished but still there.

CHAPTER 2

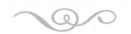

The New Face of Cancer

About EIGHT MONTHS AFTER my operation, I bumped into Dr. Luders, of all people, as he was about to board a plane in Cleveland. We were both traveling on business, a remarkable fact given the circumstances of our last encounter in the operating room. I think we were both a bit startled by the sight of each other. I broke the silence by asking him again if that passage he had had me read made any sense. I was hoping he would not say yes. Instead he laughed just as he had in the operating room and left it a mystery, which it remains to this day. But one thing was no mystery: I was speaking just fine.

After walking away from my conversation with Dr. Luders, it struck me how blessed I was to be walking through the airport, less than a year after my life-threatening surgery, with many successful cycles of chemotherapy under my belt, and fully engaged in my work. At that point I had just taken on the job of president of the American Red Cross, a position I accepted in the midst of my cancer journey with the support of my family and doctors; in fact, I encouraged the selection committee to have a chat with them as well. Would I have had the ability or the confidence to have made such a move, to return to everyday normalcy, even to schlep down the seemingly endless concourse of Cleveland-Hopkins Airport had I been diagnosed just a few years before? Unlikely. Would I have been back in the full swing of my personal life? No way. And as you will see in the pages ahead, there are many reasons for that.

A New Day

Cancer used to be viewed as a certain death sentence, and that was exactly how I viewed my prognosis on that night in 1999. But nowadays we have a new outlook on cancer, and it's a veritable sea change. Though struggling with invasive cancer can be terrifying and at times discouraging, we are beginning to turn the corner in our fight against the disease. Look at the advances in research and technology that help us diagnose and pinpoint the location of tumors and their extent. Witness the vast array of new and effective methods that limit the damage and side effects of treatment. And see virtually everywhere the increasing number of cancer survivors, 10 million in this country alone, who now view their condition as cured, or as chronic and controlled rather than as fatal, and who can miraculously resume their lives within days of an operation or treatment. For most on cancer's path, it is no longer the end of life but the beginning of life's challenging next stage.

Let me give you one of many examples. I know of a middle-aged man who was recently diagnosed with bladder cancer. Rather than refer him to hospice workers or end-of-life specialists, as the patient's mood might have indicated, his doctor told him matter-of-factly, "Look, you need to find a good urologist you really like, because you're going to be with him for the rest of your life." That advice sums up the new reality of cancer for growing numbers of patients. The battle with cancer will be a longer haul, but in this case a longer battle means a longer life, with better overall long-term prospects. In fact, in a matter of months this man had already had two successful outpatient surgeries to remove cancer from his bladder, and with each surgery he was back at work the day after and home on time to see his wife and kids. This is but one of many examples of the breakthroughs in how we understand and treat cancer. Instead of thinking, as I confess I did for a while, *This is my dying time*, cancer patients today can and should be thinking, *Every day and every moment will be a living time*. With the accelerating pace of today's cancer research, these moments translate into ever-new opportunities for treatment, remission, and cure.

But public knowledge often lags behind scientific progress, and even medical personnel, who ought to know better, can be dispiriting. Well-meaning people, often those who don't really know you or your circumstance, may overwhelm you with probing questions. Sometimes friends or colleagues convey a sense of doom and gloom when you yourself are trying to be upbeat, or subtly send the vibes that you and your illness are past history. Protecting patients and their families from discouraging backseat driving is one reason for the sacred trust of privacy between physician and patient. New doctors still swear to this trust every year when they take the ancient Oath of Hippocrates, and that means privacy for your medical records, too.

As I found out, not everyone with access to private medical information abides by this oath. In a matter of days after my diagnosis, my illness was outed, with my affliction hitting the wires, the academic gossip sheets, and the front pages of the local papers. I was later told that word seeped out of the operating room that "things did not look good for Dr. Healy," and that dire statement, if it was ever uttered, became grimmer with each retelling. A reporter even called my husband's office to confirm with Kathy Vaughn, his assistant, that I had died. Kathy, whom I'd known for years, had a good chuckle with me over that one as we recited almost in unison the Mark Twain quip that "reports of my death are greatly exaggerated." Less amusing was the run on the computerized parts of my medical record, which were called up by dozens of unauthorized rubber-neckers at the Clinic (something that would be a violation of law under today's privacy rules). I ignored most of these tacky intrusions, but it was impossible to ignore some fallout that neither my husband nor I had anticipated. This involved our girls.

Marie was shaken by the dreary medical gossip about her mother. Her friends and teachers gave her lots of support, and she was proud to report that I was now on the roster of names of people who would be getting special prayers from those who prayed at the school's chapel. But she didn't want me to find out about her struggles with stories that seemed to contradict what we had been telling her at home. I found out accidentally when I came across an e-mail she'd sent to a schoolmate, whom I'll call Melissa, in which she pleaded: "Please, Melissa, stop saying to everyone that my mom will lose all her hair and die anyway." Her friend had been innocently repeating these facts based on the authority of her own doctor-dad, who knew nothing about my case or me. Bartlett, too, was afraid to tell me that she had her own gloomy e-mails that cast my fate as "inoperable." Hey, even I didn't know what was ahead for me; how could these casual onlookers all be so sure? But my husband's unyielding optimism kept assuring us that we would lick this. And whether or not time was to prove the chatterers wrong, it made me think a lot more about the etiquette of cancer, another subject I'll discuss later. But lessons in etiquette would not be needed were people only to imagine that they were that patient or part of that family, or, for that matter, if they were to learn more about medicine's current march on cancer.

The new era of cancer detection and treatment is vastly more positive than most people think. And as you will see, the concept of cure is taking on a different meaning. The old doomsday paradigms are still with us, as our daughters found out early on, but they are gradually giving way to a new and bolder perspective on cancer.

This emerging perspective demands big-league changes in how we approach the cancer war and in what we as doctors and laypeople alike imagine cancer to be.

Let's acknowledge the worst. Yes, cancer is in our history and in our biology. Yes, it makes a huge claim on human life, with over half a million people in the United States carried off by the disease each year, most of them in the prime of their lives. Cancer is the biggest killer of our children and of those between the ages of forty-five and eighty-five, dwarfing the number of lives lost to heart disease or stroke in that older age group. These numbers are the very ones that make us all one on the cancer frontier, in arms before a very bad hombre.

That's the scary news, the bad news. But on the other side of the scale, there is something else to bring us together, and with passion: most people today survive their cancers and live full lives thereafter. Early diagnosis and better treatment have swelled the ranks of cancer survivors. Advances in molecular biology and human genetics have thoroughly altered notions of the complex genesis of the disease. They also point toward a wider range of options that is making treatment for many cancers more tailored and effective and, in some cases, less daunting. And as we come to understand the complex array of molecular patterns that underlie seemingly similar tumors, we are seeing the dawn of a more individualized approach to therapy and, by definition, a more personal and private one.

The Heart's Promise

The cancer experience can learn from the heart. I chose cardiology as my specialty back in the 1970s because of its vibrant promise based on an explosion of new developments sweeping a field that had had, before then, little to offer its patients. Not unlike cancer today, heart attacks were the health terror of most of the twentieth century. A heart attack was close to a death sentence, with good reason. Half of those who had attacks never made it to the hospital, dying suddenly and unexpectedly, and barely half of those who got to the hospital ever made it home again. Those lucky enough to survive often withdrew from life and became "cardiac cripples," as much because of their grim prognosis and their own psychological unease about resuming normal activity as because of true cardiac disability.

Cardiac catheterization, CPR, electrical defibrillators, pacemakers, coronary care units, congenital heart or valve surgery, coronary bypass procedures, angioplasty, cardiac transplantation—these innovations all have transformed what it means to be someone at risk for heart disease. Hand in hand with them came a stream of cardiac drugs to treat arrhythmias, reduce blood pressure or cholesterol, control heart failure, thin the blood, and interrupt or limit the damage of heart attacks. Another lifesaving development was the identification of coronary risk factors such as elevated cholesterol, high blood pressure, smoking, and obesity, all of which could be modified to decrease the risk of developing the disease or to slow its progress.

Science in the laboratory and at the bedside drove these advances that have made heart disease an understandable as well as a preventable and controllable problem. Coronary catheterization, a monumental innovation developed by cardiologist Mason Sones more than forty years ago, enabled physicians and scientists to grasp the underlying nature of coronary disease and its impact on the heart of individual patients. With this procedure, the catheter, a long spaghetti-sized hollow tube, is threaded from the arm or the groin into the aorta and then selectively into the small-caliber coronary arteries that branch off to deliver blood to the heart. With the coronary arteries lit up by a special dye called contrast material, the coronary angiogram creates a detailed black-and-white motion picture of the heart. Barely twenty years later, this innovation led to balloon catheters that could open up the blockages directly; later, stents were devised to keep the treated vessels open.

That a catheter could even be placed inside the human heart, much less threaded into its coronary arteries, was an awesome notion. It brought the 1956 Nobel Prize to the cardiac physiologists André Frédéric Cournand, Werner Forssmann, and Dickinson

Richards. Mason Sones received the Lasker Award, an American award often viewed as a precursor to the Nobel; had he lived longer, he might have seen that honor as well. Today we take these procedures for granted. Yet it wasn't so long ago that for cardiologists who were dealing with ailing patients on a daily basis, it seemed as if such medical discoveries were coming at glacial speed.

But think about this: it took thirty to forty years to control a disease that had caused four millennia of misery. And it was done without curing the underlying disease of atherosclerosis, but rather by containing it through a reduction of risk factors and a cast of new drugs, all based on a sturdy foundation of scientific discovery about the ways of normal hearts and those that fail. The relatively new concept of secondary prevention—in which the progress of a disease is interrupted by healthy behaviors and innovative medicines such as those for blood pressure and cholesterol control—was born in cardiovascular medicine. Keeping the atherosclerotic process in check with age-old drugs such as aspirin and new ones such as the statins is now commonplace. Heart-healthy behaviors are part of our vocabulary. Preventive cardiology may be the youngest of the medical disciplines, and it is one that can only inspire other domains of medicine—such as oncology.

Look at the many people around you, be they friends, family members, or acquaintances, or look from afar at the likes of Betty Ford, Larry King, and Bill Clinton. Their hearts were starved of oxygen by nearly choked-off coronary arteries, yet they emerged from these treatments unscathed to become healthy and energetic veterans of the disease. This is the very same disease that fifty years ago made former president Dwight Eisenhower face the relentless unchecked progression of his coronary blockages that incapacitated him after he left the White House.

In the pages ahead you will see close up how the accelerating genomic revolution has the same power to decipher many human cancers that heart catheters have had in the understanding and control of the many faces of heart disease. No question, cancer is more complex, more difficult, and more varied in its presentation than heart disease. But this war is winnable, because we finally, at long last, have the right tools. The sciences most needed to solve heart disease—microscopic pathology, physiology, biochemistry, and physics—were available early in the twentieth century. The scientific disciplines for unraveling cancer's mysteries—human genomics, proteomics, molecular biology, cell biology—emerged later in the twentieth century and early in the twenty-first, as did the innovations that brought us high-speed mathematical computations, bioinformatics, microchips, robotics, and nanotechnology, all weapons in the war against cancer.

When Richard Nixon declared that war in 1971, the world was a much different place. We were in a protracted war in Vietnam, and our cold war confrontation with the Soviet Union had created an all-or-nothing, wipe-out-or-be-wiped-out mentality. Since then, the landscape has changed, and so have the rules of engagement. Though its imagery is still ugly, today's war against cancer more closely resembles the war on terrorism, where intelligence is as important as bombs, and where localized threats in the form of rogue states and individual terror cells can be targeted and neutralized when properly detected.

That's why this war is taking so blasted long. Some are exhausted by the wait and the many unkept promises, and think we may even be losing. They point out that even though we have had over thirty years of intensive research and improved methods of treatment, the annual death toll for cancer has barely budged relative to the dramatic decline in the death rate from heart disease over that same time. But I do believe that we are at a tipping point in this war, and that the cancer field is now approaching the stage where cardiology was several decades ago. That said, this is the time for rekindling the same sense of urgency that led to the founding of the National Cancer Institute in 1937 and Nixon's official declaration of the war on cancer, and to have the faith to persevere with the talent, energy, and resources that tomorrow's successes demand.

Of Science and Faith

I've always had faith. Faith that tomorrow will be better than today. Faith that what is wrong will be righted. Faith in people and their heroism. Faith in medicine and science. And faith that there is something sacred way beyond our reach that drives our search to do better and be better. Whatever any one physician's personal beliefs might be, and however solidly grounded in science and skepticism our profession must be, there is an immutable spiritual core to the care of the patient that transcends both. And from it stems a quiet reverence for the sick that was expressed simply and memorably by the late Dr. George Crile Jr., a cancer surgeon at the Cleveland Clinic, in his 1955 book *Cancer and Common Sense*: "No physician, sleepless and worried about a patient, can return to the hospital in the midnight hours without feeling the importance of his faith. The dim corridor is silent; the doors are closed. At the end of the corridor in the glow of the desk lamp, the nurse watches over those who sleep or lie lonely and waiting behind closed doors. No physician entering the hospital in these quiet hours can help feeling that the medical institution of which he is a part is in essence religious, that it is built on trust. No physician can fail to be proud that he is part of his patient's faith."

My own experience with patients has given me a profound respect for the power of a patient's faith, in whatever form it takes, to influence the course of his or her illness and perhaps the length of life, which is hard to prove by scientific method. Most certainly, however, it can better the quality of life. Working with the critically ill, or being ill, inevitably stirs the spirit to think about what binds us all together and what might lie beyond our own mortality. On this, surely, we cannot escape our roots.

I grew up steeped in religious faith, though I have to confess I'm what some would call a fallen Catholic—a fate, in retrospect, that I've flirted with for as long as I could read. Growing up next door to St. Patrick's Church and attending the parish grammar school imbued me with religion, yet kindled a rebellious streak for science and thought that was sometimes at odds with doctrine. Our quiet street was tucked into a semi-industrial area of Long Island City in Queens, a staunchly devout Italian immigrant neighborhood that made the parish name, and my family's Irish roots, local oddities. But on 28th Street oddity was okay, as the common denominator was a lust for education fueled by the many parents who had missed out themselves. This ethic no doubt contributed to my becoming a hopeless but proud geek. Reading, reading, and more reading was also our family's religion, and those books regularly got me in hot water with the nuns, particularly when I was caught reading a few authors that were on the banned list—such as Tolstoy.

I spent most of my savings on books, too, and one of my prized acquisitions was a little red prayer book. I discovered it in a Catholic bookstore in Manhattan, billed as a companion to the breviary that I could see the priests reading as they walked almost daily in the schoolyard right next to our house. What a find! I was sure it contained all their secret prayers. What it actually contained were selected psalms from the Old Testament, and they were a discovery. At the time we Catholics were discouraged from reading the Bible directly; we were supposed to stick to the catechism instead. But here I had an insider's view of the Bible through the psalms, which soon became my prayer book.

Somehow over the years I lost track of my precious psalm book. To my great astonishment, just after I fell ill, my mom brought me that little book, which she had kept tucked away all these years, still in the dusty brown paper I'd wrapped it in for protection. On the inside cover, I had written my name, address, and the date, which made me thirteen years old at the time. This red prayer book was a bit like my daughter Marie's blankie and ducky, the simple treasures you connect with deeply when you are very young and that still bring you comfort when you are grown up. What made Mom's discovery even more special was that the frayed red ribbon marker opened the worn little book to the page containing the 29th Psalm (the 30th Psalm in most versions of the Bible). It was headed "A Prayer in Time of Sickness." Mom and I both wondered—was this somehow providential? Scientists are not supposed to think that way. But she had never opened the book, and I could not remember when I had seen it last. So we were both quite happy to smile and take its message as a good sign for things to come.

This psalm is not a simple plea for salvation, by the way. Rather, it's a prayer of thanks for having been healed, added to a not-so-subtle negotiation with God about why He was right to have done so. The psalmist argues that it was too soon to be cast into the pits, and questions what good that would have done anyway. "Shall the dust praise thee?" he asks. I suspect it was not just the thanksgiving or the medical theme that drew me to this psalm years ago. It was the bartering. I had already made celestial negotiation a veritable art form, directed toward my major goal in life: doing well in school so that I could go to college.

I figured out a secret weapon for academic success: a hefty group of unnamed and unknown saints who I knew would intercede on my behalf with the Big Guy, because I had already interceded for them. The nuns had told us that a mass with Holy Communion, and a rosary added on to close the deal, would lift a poor soul languishing in purgatory up and through the pearly gates. Living next door to the church, it was easy for me to go to 6:30 mass during the week, where I prayed specifically for scholarly souls. If I had a math exam, I asked for the ascent of a math teacher; a science test, a biologist; for history, a historian; and religion, some smart nun, at least if the lot of them weren't already in heaven. Somehow it worked. My psalm book, so lovingly protected by Mom over the years, gave me many moments of solace during my cancer journey. But I was delighted to find a new saint to accompany me as well. An Italian, no less.

Peregrine Laziosi is the patron saint of cancer patients. He is a little-known saint from Forlì, Italy—a regular sort of guy, hardworking and pious with a restless past. At age sixty he came down with cancer and seemed doomed. But the evening before his leg was to be amputated he prayed all night, and by morning the tumor had mysteriously and spontaneously disappeared. For many years thereafter, he devoted himself to good works, dying in his eighties of natural causes in 1345. In 1726 Benedict XIII, who as pope remained devoted to his friarly work by visiting the sick and dying, canonized Peregrine as a saint, undoubtedly seeing the need for him.

My interest in St. Peregrine was less about believing in saints and more about spiritual inspiration. That's what saints, mere mortal souls, are about. Who does not grasp the charity of a Mother Teresa, or the courage of Joan of Arc, or the educational devotion of Mother Elizabeth Ann Seton, the first American-born person to become a saint? Even in their most secular form, saints teach us by example how to walk the right way, and offer a personal refuge to those wearied by a similar plight. They show that, at heart and over time, life is a common journey.

I was drawn to Peregrine because he was not a martyr killed by the sword or burned at the stake but a heroic figure with a miraculous spontaneous remission of his deadly cancer. In that, St. Peregrine's way is one of faith with a scientific twist. It zeroes in on the single most important mystery of cancer, the secret of remission, which is the goal of cancer therapy.

At the very least, the annals of cancer are to be read with humility. Medically unexpected or even spontaneous remissions—however rare—tell us that cancer can be cured by means that are still unknown to us. If even one human being is saved, it could be many. The book of knowledge on the complex genetic and molecular instructions that can make our human cells go bad, and then reverse their fortunes, is just now being written. When it is completed it will tell Peregrine's story as well as ours. And along the way, Peregrine reminds us not to undervalue the spiritual side of our humanness, which gives us the strength to deal with life's greatest challenges.

In the early days of my life with cancer I felt a haunting grayness, a feeling that I was only half on this earth. The best of me seemed to be slipping away in some vague but powerful undertow, taking with it my confidence. This was something that I was not prepared for, even though working with life-threatening illness was my profession. I would have to learn, just as every patient does, by walking. The path I stumbled along had its dark times, but also its moments of joy. Some events seemed to turn the tide of my disease; and then others brought major setbacks. In these pages I will spare you full details of my medical history, in part to honor the few shreds of privacy I've managed to retain, but also to keep the focus on what is universal in our common cancer journey and on how we find the courage we need to prevail.

As I look back on the years since I first faced my own cancer, I think mostly about those I love. Marie is in college, my precious confidant with a psychology bent; Bart, with an advanced degree in national security, is happily working in Washington, D.C., soon to be married to a wonderful fellow named Adam. Our grandson Wyatt has a brother named Henry. I'm back to looking after Mom. We have lost, so unexpectedly, my dear Michele and Nonie, but they fill my heart in their loving and inspiring way. As for Fred, his trees are growing lush and strong in the great outdoors. Not long ago, he and I again watched an Oscar De La Hoya fight on television, and this time the only one knocked out was his opponent. Fred and I toasted this fact. Every day there are these kinds of battles happily being won by cancer patients and their families. And to us all, every day is a celebration.

For me and, I believe, for most others, what ultimately gets us through is a simple formula: love beyond ourselves, plus our mental and physical labors, plus modern medicine—a medicine that's not perfect, not there yet, but well on its way. The journey itself is quintessentially personal. Know what you want, and what you most value. Read and consult. Negotiate hard. Have faith. And think of the closing words of a letter hastily scribbled to me by Bartlett on the eve of my cancer surgery: "I will never give up hope. I will not let you stop fighting—and I do believe in miracles."

PART TWO

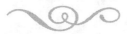

How Cancer
Comes to Be

*The capacity to blunder slightly is the real
marvel of DNA. Without this special
attribute, we would still be anaerobic
bacteria and there would be no music.*

—*The Medusa and the Snail*,
Lewis Thomas, M.D.

CHAPTER 3

Anatomy of Cancer

HOW CAN THIS BE?" "Why me?" The sudden jolt that overtakes you when you are told you have cancer is followed by sheer puzzlement. In an instant, your mind races in search of what you might have done to cause this; it scans the branches of the family tree for others who might have shared the same fate. It does not matter how schooled you are in the ways of science and medicine—the shock and confusion are there. I've seen it in my loved ones, in patients, in the teary eyes of parents embracing their otherwise perfect child. And I've felt it myself.

How and why are the kinds of questions the healthy avoid asking; perhaps it's a wishful denial that cancer will ever draw near enough to matter. But denial and avoidance have no place in a world in which close to half of us will face this diagnosis—and all will hold the hand of someone who experiences cancer. Everyone has a stake in the why of this disease.

Cancer comes with the human condition. The exquisite genetic complexity that makes us who we are is at the same time our Achilles' heel, vulnerable to genetic mishaps. Cancer may start out as a few chemical blunders deep within the nucleus of the cell, but it gradually rewrites a patient's genetic code, almost becoming a new lifeform. It is only now that sophisticated molecular and genomic technology have let us decode the many DNA changes that lead to the hundreds of different forms of cancer. Though the disease has many different labels and can appear in virtually all tissues, there are specific traits that provide cancer's malignant force, whatever the individual pattern of gene changes happens to be. Focusing with scientific ferocity on these traits and how they come to be has made (and will continue to make) this disease less mysterious and will ultimately force its secrets to give way. For there is no reason why cancer should triumph; fully exposed, it proves to have numerous points of vulnerability.

Benign or Malignant?

What is cancer? In the simplest terms it is a growth in the body, and of the body, that has no purpose. It takes up space, and it wastes the energies it steals from the organs and tissues in which it arises. Descriptions of cancer are as old as recorded time. An Egyptian papyrus dating from 1600 B.C. portrays cancer and physicians' efforts to destroy it with knives, burns, and potions. Inca mummies with cancer have been unearthed from the pre-Columbian period in Peru, within a few hundred years of the time that Hippocrates, on the other side of the globe, cared for patients with cancers, attributing them to an excess of black bile, one of the four bodily humors of Greek medicine. From what we can tell, tumors of ancient time were very much as we see them today, except they were bigger and more advanced— our ancestors had almost no options for defeating them. In A.D. 30, the Roman physician Aulus Cornelius Celsus, who penned an eight-volume work on medicine, coined the term *tumor*, meaning "swelling." Advanced growths are warm and painful and can ulcerate through the skin with a look not so different from the infected wounds that were a common affliction of his day. So it's no surprise that Celsus tied *tumor*, swelling, to three other traits we know to be linked to inflammation: *rubor, calor,* and *dolor*—that is, redness, heat, and pain. By his definition, a tumor could be either an abscess or a new growth.

Though Celsus was ahead of his time in linking tumor to inflammation, we now reserve the term *tumor* only for a neoplasm, or a new growth. But Celsus's advance in understanding was limited, and ancient theories dominated medical thinking about cancer into modern times—the black bile theory persisted for almost two thousand years. In fact, the situation didn't start to change until the advent of one of the most powerful medical tools of all time: the microscope. Invented in the late 1600s by Antony van Leeuwenhoek, this instrument opened the world of cells and tissues to the human eye, just as the telescope revealed the distant heavens.

As is still the case today, it took just such a technological advance to finally challenge long-outmoded medical notions of health and disease. The application and spread of technology was slow back then, though, and it was 200 more years before the microscope was finally applied to the study of cancer. With the instrument's power came the discovery that neoplasms were distinct masses of microscopic cells, laid out in strange and disorderly fashion. This microscopic portrait gave physicians enough information to lump tumors into one of two forms: benign or malignant. The tumors that stopped growing looked much like normal organ cells under the microscope and were benign. Malignant tumors, in contrast, which grew relentlessly and led to skin ulceration and debilitation if not death, bore markedly less resemblance to normal cells; they often had a wild, frenzied look microscopically. This distinction was the first major advance in cancer medicine in almost 2,000 years, and it still holds.

Today, we're in the middle of a technological revolution every bit as transforming as the microscope. Cancer has its origins within the DNA of individual cells, and to peer there requires the modern-day tools of molecular and cell biology. With the molecular technologies that now exist to explore the human genome, we have the power and the speed to intercept the orders sent from the cell's nucleus to create the structure of the cells and tissues we see under the microscope. This allows us to sort out the many complex forms of tumors, benign and cancerous.

Fortunately, most tumors are benign, merely lazy lumps of slowly growing cells. Though they may look like their neighboring cells, they are freeloaders, doing little or no work. To be sure, benign tumors can be life-threatening, but mostly for mechanical reasons. For example, benign brain tumors can squeeze healthy cells into dysfunction because their mass builds pressure inside the rigid and nonexpandable skull. The heart, which rarely struggles with cancer, is prone to a particular kind of benign tumor called a myxoma, which dangles on a stalk inside the heart's chambers and when large and floppy enough can block blood flow. Well known to women are the benign tumors of the uterus. Most of the time these uterine fibroids cause no problems, but if they get large and cause severe pain and bleeding, a hysterectomy may be required.

Benign tumors are known more for all the bad things they *don't* do. They don't grow fast or without limit, they don't destroy the hardworking neighbor cells, and they don't peel off and spread, or metastasize, to other organs. Benign tumors stop growing on their own, and sometimes disappear spontaneously. For all the fear and horror their first appearance can cause, these are the innocent ones. And that's what prompts the first question that comes to mind when one is told about a tumor: "Is it benign or malignant?"

Cells Gone Wild

One thing you learn in medical school is that you have to understand what's healthy before you can understand what's happening in disease. Healthy, normal cells—some trillions strong that make up each of our bodies—are a disciplined lot. They are forever locked into a tightly choreographed cycle of growth, development, hard work, and quiet death. Individual cells work together as part of a team, developing the special characteristics that make them a functioning unit of tissue and then part of an organ system that serves the whole body's needs.

Central to this organization is the ability of the genome (present in its entirety in every bodily cell) to selectively turn on some genes and silence others in order to fashion the specialty cells that make up our tissues and organs and their vital functions. For example, a certain set of genes produces the mature heart cells that are able to contract continually, while another set produces very different-looking and -behaving nerve cells, the squid-like neurons of the brain and spinal cord crafted for communication. Another mix of genes makes a liver cell work as a chemical processing and detoxifying plant, and a kidney cell cleanse the blood and balance the body's salt and water.

This well-defined specialization is the result of a process that begins early in embryonic life as primitive stem cells become mature and differentiated. In the laboratory, isolated cultures of stem cells can reproduce indefinitely and, if properly stimulated, have the ability to turn into any kind of cell. Scientists are interested in that potential to be able to grow cells to replace a patient's damaged ones. But once normal stem cells turn into specialty cells in the body, they don't turn back, and they also lose the ability to grow endlessly.

Perhaps our bodies' cells have taken a page from the world of bees, where the vast majority are organized into teams of workers that shun reproductive activities, spending all their energies on the constant, highly technical efforts of building and sustaining the hive. In cancer, the discipline and teamwork of the body's specialized "worker cells" is subverted. Cancer cells originate within specific organ systems, but they pull away from their team, abandon any obligation for work, and shift their energies to endless and frenetic reproduction. The beautiful teamwork becomes chaos in the process.

A visible characteristic of a malignant growth is that it looks less and less like the normal tissue in which it began to grow. You may see cancer cells referred to as "undifferentiated," which means they lack the defining characteristics of mature, healthy cells. In cancer parlance they are "anaplastic," with irregular shapes, distorted internal cell structures, and large, dense, angry nuclei caught in the midst of doubling or tripling their chromosomes as they pursue hyperactive growth. Sometimes cancer cells are so primitive that even a skilled pathologist studying the tissue under the microscope can't identify its cellular origins—whether it is breast, liver, colon, or prostate.

It's customary for pathologists to grade tumors based on their visible state of normality or differentiation when viewed under the microscope. The verdict "well differentiated" is usually good news for cancer patients; it means that the tumor is apt to grow more slowly. This is the lowest grade, or grade I, cancer. As one goes up on a scale of I to IV, grade II and III tumors are progressively less differentiated (i.e., they look less normal). The highest-grade and most primitive-looking tumors are grade IV, and they tend to be faster-growing.

But remember, grade is only a microscopic take on an isolated sample of a tumor. And it is different from stage, which is measured on another scale of 0 to IV that is used by oncologists to indicate whether a cancer has spread. Stage 0 means that cancer cells have not invaded at all; stage IV indicates they have metastasized to distant parts of the body (see page 60). Grade, stage, and the specific anatomic site of origin of the tumor (such as breast or colon) form a common classification system that helps doctors compare tumors, and determine the type and intensity of treatment.

What makes cancer so complex is that it's detected in different grades and stages, but also in as many varieties as there are specialty cells and organs in the body. While they may share common origins and characteristics, cancers exhibit a range of forms and behaviors that rivals the exuberant diversity of animals in the wild. And as different species, they are classified to be better understood. In the broadest classification, cancers are lumped into solid, soft tissue, and liquid forms.

The solid cancers, which include the most common cancers that affect humans, are called carcinomas. Carcinomas arise in the specialized epithelial cells that cover the body and line organs. For example, they make up skin; line the mouth, the gut, and the air passages of the lung; and form the ducts of the breast and prostate. The ducts in the breast, prostate, and colon are specialized epithelial cells that secrete compounds such as milk and mucus.

Liquid cancers are those that affect the blood and lymphatic systems, and include the many forms of leukemia, the lymphomas, and multiple myeloma. The relatively rare sarcomas are the soft tissue cancers that involve the body's support structures—fibrous tissue, bone, and muscle. Cancers of the brain and central nervous system fall into their own class.

All together there are about two hundred different types of cancer. Despite this variety, there are common principles and behaviors that make cancer one as well as many. By getting inside cancer cells and decoding their DNA, scientists have learned that no matter how diverse, these cells all go ugly in pretty much the same way.

Cancer as a Disease of Our DNA

Rocks don't get cancer, but complex life-forms, driven by a self-replicating genetic program, do. The inanimate rock may weather with time, grow mossy, discolor, and be shattered to oblivion, but it will never get cancer, simply because it lacks DNA. Cancer directly changes the DNA code, thereby altering the cell's fundamental identity and behavior and forever changing its future. The inborn genetic code of the normal cell is progressively modified in cancerous clones so that it no longer contributes to the well-being of the body. Rather, with a design set by their own altered DNA, the cancer clones become survival specialists at the expense of the organ and body in which they originated. These clones carry on only because they hijack a wide range of everyday, normal cell processes, allowing for unrestrained growth and invasion. The cancer genome has an overdose of some genes and an absence or paucity of others. In some cases, genes and chromosomes are broken and refigured into entirely new creations.

READING THE BOOK OF LIFE: *THE HUMAN GENOME*

Chromosomes are like spools for genetic information—a convenient way for cells to package the extraordinarily long, thin molecules that encode their genes, without getting them all tangled up. Each chromosome is made of two thread-like strands of the genetic material, DNA or deoxyribonucleic acid, which spiral around each other in a regular pattern called a double helix. Each strand of DNA is a single molecule, built up like a chain composed of repeating subunits, called nucleotides. Nucleotides come in four molecular types: adenine (A), thymine (T), guanine (G), and cytosine (C). Depending on their order—or sequence—these four "letters" spell out a series of different "words" along the DNA strand. Each word is just three nucleotides long, and each represents a single instruction, either spelling out the genetic code for a particular amino acid (amino acids are proteins' building blocks) or acting as a punctuation mark, telling the cellular machinery when and where to start and stop reading. The three-letter words, called codons, are further sequenced into "sentences" and "paragraphs" that tell a complete story—that is, they provide all of the information needed to make a specific protein. These functional units are called genes.

Humans have some 25,000 genes (21,000 confirmed and another 4,000 presumed), scattered across twenty-three pairs of chromosomes—one member of each pair from each parent. Each chromosome pair has its own characteristic size and microscopic shape, though almost all take on the form of an impressionistic X, with two adjacent arms shorter than the other two. Together, the 25,000 genes make up the human genome. With the exception of red blood cells, which lack DNA, every cell in the human body contains the entire human genome. But only a few of these genes are actively being read, or "expressed," at any given time in any particular cell.

When a gene is activated, it forms a short-lived messenger molecule, RNA or ribonucleic acid, in its mirror image, like a photographic negative. This RNA template in turn translates the genetic code into a functioning protein. Proteins are the heavy-lifters of the cellular world; some, like elastin and collagen, give organs and tissues their strength and flexibility. Others, the enzymes, work as tiny chemical factories, breaking down food, for example, or manufacturing fats and carbohydrates. A group of generally small proteins, the hormones, works as molecular messengers, delivering physiological command and control information throughout the body. The sum total of proteins produced by active genes is called the proteome.

It is this proteome that determines our traits: what we look like, how our organs function and work together, and even some aspects of temperament and nascent talents such as an operatic voice or ability with math. The genes are important, of course—without them there could be no proteins—but if a gene is silent and does not translate into its protein, it might as well not be there. As we will see, genes, together with the complex cellular machinery that controls how and when they are expressed, play a critical role in resistance or susceptibility to many diseases, including cancer.

Long before we had any knowledge of genes, scientists connected cancer and chromosomes. A century ago, Theodor Boveri, a German biologist who had already made a name for himself by describing normal chromosomes, began to study cancer cells under the microscope. There he could see chromosomes that had gone haywire—broken, distorted in shape, doubled or tripled up. In what was surely a eureka moment, he made the connection that cancer must be caused by abnormal and unstable chromosomes. This was a huge discovery, and one that has held up well over time.

But Boveri's theory had unsettling exceptions: not all cancer cells displayed the visibly wild chromosomal distortions. It was not until scientists had the wherewithal to identify the many smaller and more subtle distortions hiding within the strands of DNA that Boveri's insight was validated. He was on the right track but just didn't have the technology to get down to the gene level to prove it.

Because cancer is in our genes, does that mean that all cancer is inherited? The answer is no. Some people are born with cancer susceptibility traits that have been passed on through their family—that is, through the germ cells better known as sperm and egg. (I'll discuss this more in Chapter 4.) But before we jump too quickly to blame our ancestors, it should be made clear that most of the DNA mistakes that trigger and sustain cancer occur because of the very processes of living and aging and interacting with an ever-changing world. Life requires that our cells copy themselves to give birth to new generations of cells—first as we develop and grow to adulthood, and also to replace dead or decrepit cells as we age. And in the complex process of copying DNA, mistakes can and do happen, whether inadvertently or as the result of chemical assault, infectious disease, or other interactions with an often hostile environment. These are the mutations, slowly accumulating over time, that occur within somatic cells (which make up the organs of our bodies) but do not pass their genetic information on to future generations. This explains why cancers most often attack people as they grow older.

READING THE BOOK OF LIFE:
CELL REPRODUCTION

When cells divide, or clone themselves—whether as part of normal, controlled growth or as a result of a cancerous binge—the process starts in the cell's nucleus. There, the tightly twisted resting chromosomes relax as all the DNA along all forty-six strands (two for each chromosome) is copied, nucleotide by nucleotide. It takes four to eight hours to accomplish this task, and another hour or two for the cell to proofread its work and repair any mistakes in the new DNA sequence before the cell divides in two. If you imagine this process happening at this very moment throughout your body, repeated billions of times each day throughout a lifetime, you get a hint of just how easy it might be for one of those gene copies to go wrong—a misspelling, a deletion, a duplication, a mixed-up gene swapping—and set the deadly march of cancer into motion.

There are at least four different ways that genes change on the road to cancer. It's worth understanding these mechanisms, because they explain many puzzles, such as why someone can inherit a cancer gene but never get the disease, and what makes strategies for prevention and treatment really work—or not.

Changing a Gene's Chemical Structure: Mutations

Mutations change the chemical sequence of the DNA; often, a mutation is a seemingly minor change, a little misspelling here or there within a gene. Most misspellings have no consequence; others, depending largely on where they fall, can alter the entire function of the gene, making it more powerful, making it different, or silencing it altogether. For the most part the mutations that have accumulated and survived over generations are the ones that create the marvelous diversity of our human family and the individuality of each person, such as the color of one's eyes or the curl of one's hair.

Mutations, in fact, occur all the time in nature; this was the idea at the core of Charles Darwin's theory of evolution. Whether in the beaks of Darwin's Galapagos finches, in the physical traits of *Homo sapiens*, or in the cells of a burgeoning cancer, those mutations most fit for survival—for growing and dominating—prevail. There is one huge difference, of course, between normal evolution and cancer development. The mutations that change normal traits get passed on because they help the person or animal survive in the context of their external environment. Mutations that make cancer help only the cancer cells survive, enabling them to flourish in the body's internal environment at the expense of normal cells.

As a group, genes that have mutated in a way that makes them a party to cancer development are called oncogenes. (*Onco-*, meaning "mass," derives from the Greek.) And understanding that mutations play a role in the development of cancer is central to cancer prevention. We have learned, for example, to avoid chemical or radiation exposures that are known to damage DNA. (See Chapter 6.)

Changing a Gene's Environment: Epigenetics

Sometimes a gene is present but an external factor interferes with its ability to translate its DNA code into action. It's not enough to have the gene; the gene has to be able to pass its orders on to the messenger molecules that in turn translate the message into the correct protein. The way DNA does this is through the messenger molecule RNA. If some external factor within the cell, or within the genome itself, throws a monkey wrench into the message transfer process, a normal gene is shut down. One example of this process is called gene methylation, in which a small fragment of a molecule (a methyl group) gloms onto a gene and literally smothers it. With its communications path cut off, the gene cannot express itself. This process, called epigenetics, is of great interest to cancer specialists since it explains why some tumors become resistant to drug treatment:

methylation silences key genes that have been helping the treatment kill off the cancer.

Sometimes it is the RNA messenger itself that turns traitor and smothers a gene into inactivity. A small RNA interference molecule (RNAi) can attach to a piece of DNA and block its ability to be expressed into a protein. Increasingly, RNAi is emerging not only as another monkey wrench that the body uses to help tweak gene expression but also as an opportunity: scientists are crafting man-made RNA interference molecules to target and shut down specific genes that are misbehaving.

Thus, modern cancer detective work searches for abnormal, absent, or overexpressed proteins as well as identifying the genes that carry their source codes. Having the DNA blueprints is not enough; you want to know exactly what proteins the genes actually deliver— or whether they deliver any proteins at all. In short, epigenetics speaks to the personal environment in which a cell lives and functions, and how that environment influences gene activity. Epigenetic differences help explain why one woman who has a gene for breast cancer never gets the disease yet her sister with the same gene has her life cut short. Genes do not work in a vacuum.

Disordering Hunks of Chromosomes: Aneuploidy

Sometimes a cancer genome arises as a result of a major chromosomal disaster of the sort Boveri first identified a hundred years ago. Called aneuploidies, these are genetic train wrecks, in which big hunks of molecular sequences along the chromosome are deleted, multiplied, or swapped with sections on other chromosomes. Unlike mutations or epigenetic changes, which are highly specific distortions of an individual gene, aneuploidy is an indiscriminate mass distortion of whole stretches of the genome all in one blow. (This form of cancer-related DNA change factored into my own tumor.)

The net effect is that hundreds or even thousands of genes are randomly added or eliminated at the same time. Deletions of the long or short arms of specific chromosomes are seen in many forms of cancer; there are also translocations, in which segments of chromosomes filled with genes are swapped between chromosomes. For example, in chronic myelogenous leukemia, one of the most common cancers of the white blood cells, the ends of chromosomes 9 and 22 are swapped. This results in an entirely new chromosome (named Philadelphia) and a new hybrid protein (called BCR-ABL) that is cancer-causing. That information helps doctors understand the nature of the cancer, and even more important, provides a target for drug therapy. A grand example of this is the blockbuster drug Gleevec (imatinib), designed specifically to target cancers that have a Philadelphia chromosome. (More on this in Chapter 10.)

Bringing New DNA in from the Outside World: Oncogenic Viruses

On rare occasions viruses carry abnormal genetic material into certain cells and contribute to cancer development. In such cases, the infecting viruses introduce their own genes into the host cell. The net result can be a novel protein that is cancer-inciting. While virus-induced cancers are fairly common in the animal world, fortunately they are uncommon in humans. The exceptions, however, are dramatic.

Among the most widespread of the cancer-causing viruses is the sexually transmitted human papillomavirus (HPV), which often causes visible genital warts. HPV is the major cause of a worldwide epidemic of cancer of the cervix. Oncogenic strains of HPV introduce alien DNA into cervical cells with nefarious effect—it inhibits two critical gene proteins that actually prevent cancer formation, including the suppressor gene *p53* (see page 56). With the protective genes inactivated, the stage is set for a stepwise progression to cervical cancer. Recognizing that the risk of cervical cancer is sexually transmitted has preventive value, particularly since two vaccines have been developed that provide almost complete immunity to the specific HPV strains that are known to be cancer connected.

Darwin's Bad Clones

It's one thing for chance or injury to alter a gene; it's quite another for a collection of these alterations to create a new and malignant life-form. But this is what happens when, in a process of rapid Darwinian selection, cell clones with ever more wild and rambunctious genes gain a survival advantage over their more disciplined and orderly parents and cousins. In this process of "clonal evolution," each successive surviving generation has the chance to intensify its survival talents. In human cancers this generally happens over years if not decades, as multiple genes must go haywire to finally make a cell clone that has mastered the most powerful skills of cancer—the secrets of both immortality and invasion. In this dynamic process the genome of the cancer cell becomes progressively more unstable.

Bert Vogelstein, a Johns Hopkins cancer researcher, has devoted his career to methodically exposing this genetic evolution in colon cancer. His laboratory showed that all forms of this cancer—whether they occur in families or develop spontaneously—have similar patterns of stepwise accumulation of mutations, originating within the lining cells of the bowel. The accumulating mutations correspond to the progression of colon cancer, from a benign but pre-cancerous polyp to a virulent, invasive tumor, with each evolving generation's mutations accounting for the nastier and nastier behavior. These discoveries offer a firm scientific rationale for finding and treating tumors early—whether the first step on the road to cancer is an inherited gene, a random occurrence, or even a virus.

The Stem Cells of Cancer

New research is also uncovering a previously hidden tumor mastermind: cancerous stem cells. Under normal circumstances we carry adult stem cells—separate and apart from the embryonic stem cells, which exist only in the very early embryo—throughout our lives as important agents of renewal and repair. They are present throughout the body, poised to spin off new specialized cells as the need arises. The adult stem cells are particularly abundant in the bone marrow, where blood cells renew themselves in a matter of days to weeks. (Not surprisingly, their cancerous transformation has long been implicated in leukemia.)

Normal adult stem cells share some qualities with cancer: under the microscope they don't look like the cells they can turn into; they can freely roam about the body, both within organs and through the lymph and blood vessels; and they can clone themselves indefinitely. Scientists have learned to identify stem cells by unique sets of surface markers, and with that technology have been able to sift out cancerous stem cells from blood samples of those with cancer, or from tumors themselves.

Research studies have shown these cells to be the tumor-initiating cells in a few types of cancer, such as leukemia, breast, and brain. Some clever experiments are pretty convincing on this: when the cancerous stem cells are isolated from tumors and then injected into special lab animals, the animals die quickly of large tumors. But cancerous cells from the same tumors *without* stem cell markers behave differently. When these cells (which make up the bulk of the tumor mass) are injected, the resulting tumors neither grow large nor kill the animals. Instead, they produce tumors that grow only to modest proportions and then peter out.

Peter Dirks and his colleagues from the University of Toronto found tumor-initiating stem cells in every brain tumor type they studied. They showed that the most aggressive and fastest-growing grade IV brain tumor, glioblastoma multiforme, had a markedly higher number of the cancerous stem cells than slower-growing forms. Thus the density of the tumor-initiating cells within a cancer may also be a measure of its aggressiveness. As you might imagine, I took particular note of these findings, because my own tumor is known to contain nests of these primitive cells. The big uncertainty for me, and for every patient who sees their tumor shrink to almost nothing, is whether lurking in the shadows is a cluster of these cancerous stem cells, quietly waiting to rise again.

It is not yet clear whether tumor-originating cells start out as stem cells or whether, in the process of becoming cancerous, mature cells devolve into primitive stem-cell-like form. Whichever it is, this concept is shaking up some of our thinking about how we find cancer—suggesting, for example, a blood test for the cells roaming in the blood. Or how we might treat it: go directly for the stem cells that initiate and propel the tumor's growth and seed its spread. Focus there, rather than on the bulk of the tumor cells, which might then fizzle out on their own.

This work may have even broader importance if Stanford University stem cell research pioneer Irving Weissman is correct. He believes that stem cells bearing cancer genomes will ultimately prove to seed all forms of cancer. And stem cell biology in general will surely help us understand and perhaps control the single most important characteristic of cancer cells: their ability to clone themselves perpetually.

CHAPTER 4

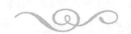

The Hubris of Immortality

A COMMON THREAT OF all cancer is its single-minded quest for its own immortality. Perpetual cloning forces cancer's ever-expanding horde of offspring cells to move into new territory at the expense of normal cells, which, hobbled by their programming to behave, can't fight off the invaders. Having lost their own reproductive skills, healthy mature cells are just pushed aside by cancer's swarming offspring.

Mortality is an essential quality of life. It distinguishes living forms from inanimate objects, people from inert matter, humans from gods. In Greek mythology, only the gods were immortal, and humans who sought this power invariably met their doom. Look at poor Asclepius, the father of medicine, a mere mortal laboring for his many patients. He was so successful in healing those on earth that god-in-chief Zeus became fearful that mortals would live forever and Hades would become depopulated. And so Asclepius met his comeuppance: he was plucked from earth and placed in the heavens as a star, destined to live forever as a minor god, a virtual inanimate object—visible and well controlled. Over the ages, other mortals—from Alexander the Great to Juan Ponce de León—have searched for immortality, without even as much success as Asclepius.

Today this ancient quest continues in the form of medical exploration. Modern immortality hunters are seeking their fountain of youth not across horizons of untamed lands and peoples but rather in the secrets of the living cell. In Asclepian tradition, "regenerative medicine" aims at replacing cells, tissues, and organs, one after another, as they show signs of decline. Some leaders in the field foresee that genetic manipulations, tissue engineering, and stem cell transplants, combined with assorted bionic tune-ups, could easily extend the human life span to 150 years. And once there, as some avid regenerists claim, why not forever? Though history tells us the human longing for everlasting life will never cease, the thought of living forever seems to me a rather dreadful one, tiring at the least—and certain to mandate the annihilation of future generations at the worst.

I should add that this line of pursuit is quite separate from the yearning of most regeneration advocates to live out a human biological life span of ninety to a hundred years, functioning well mentally and physically until the end. Eyeing human immortality as the next step after that is an entirely different matter. And we need not look too far to see the danger, for the cancer cell has mastered that madness.

Fountain of Youth

People don't age; their cells do. And that discovery about aging has brought insights into cancer's endless growth. In 1984, a team of scientists headed by Elizabeth Blackburn, now of the University of California, San Francisco, discovered what many scientists call the fountain of youth. (She won the Lasker Award for this work in 2006.) It's an enzyme called telomerase, found in the course of research being done on normal aging. Telomerase preserves and rebuilds a little piece of DNA on our chromosomes called the telomere, which functions like a timekeeper counting off the number of times any given set of chromosomes can copy itself during normal growth and reproduction.

Telomeres cap the ends of chromosomes and keep the DNA strands carrying our genes from fraying or sticking each time they duplicate themselves. This chromosome cap was first discovered in the 1930s by the Nobel laureate Barbara McClintock while at the University of Missouri at Columbia, and by Hermann Muller while at the University of Edinburgh. Subsequently it became clear that with each cell division telomeres get shorter, until they disappear. Just as the rings of a tree increase in number with age, the decreasing length of telomeres tracks the number of times—from the embryo stage on—a mature cell has copied itself. For most human cells the limit is about fifty times. When the telomere is consumed, the cell can no longer clone itself. Then its function is solely to work and be part of a community of other adult cells, aging along the way.

Telomeres are one key to human growth and aging. People born with Werner syndrome, a rare genetic disease of premature aging, have shortened telomeres that allow for just twenty doublings. Those with the disease become wrinkled and gray in their twenties; beset with such illnesses as osteoporosis, arteriosclerosis, and cataracts, they usually die in their forties. The underlying genetic defect in this disease lies within a gene that has responsibility for maintaining healthy telomeres—that is, the gene for the telomere rebuilder, telomerase.

By building back telomeres, this fountain-of-youth enzyme restores a cell's ability to clone itself. Obviously, telomerase is active in the egg and sperm, and in the rapidly developing embryo and fetus. But the enzyme is also present in adult stem cells. Think, for example, about skin, which needs to replenish the dead cells that slough off every day. When adult stem cells lying at the base of the epidermis split into two, one cell spins off as another stem cell (with telomerase) but the other is a new somatic cell, specialized to become an epidermal cell and lacking telomerase. The fresh new somatic cell can copy itself fifty or more times, thereby replenishing the dead and dying cells sloughed off the surface of the epidermis. Such genius: the new epidermal cells keep skin fresh, while the stem cell copy carries on to split in two again as needed.

This is where cancer's cleverness comes in. To grow relentlessly, the cancer genome reactivates telomerase, taking the brakes off chromosome copying. Controversy exists as to just how critical telomerase is in early cancer development. Is telomerase reactivation a consequence of the cell becoming more primitive, or is telomerase a primary cause of frenzied replication that sets cells up for mutational errors?

The aging and death of adult cells appear to be one of the body's mechanisms for preventing the harm caused by accumulated mutations. Some scientists have suggested that adult cells lose their long-term reproductive powers in order to put a limit on how many times any cell can copy its DNA, since with each duplication there is a chance for a genetic error. Capping the number of possible replications may reduce the risk of cancer that arises when mutated genes pile up. In Mother Nature's wisdom, the adult cell ages as it copies itself, perishing before self-inflicted errors can threaten the entire organism. So strongly does she feel that way, nature has additionally programmed a poison pill into the genome to kill off cells that have really messed up their DNA copies—another natural control that cancer must thwart in order to thrive.

Subverting Poison Pills

Apoptosis is a Greek word that refers to the falling of petals from a dying flower or the autumn leaves from a tree. In 1972, this poetic name was given to the process of natural and purposeful cell death.

It describes the body's easy and systematic way of eliminating cells that are no longer needed or too old or damaged to do their jobs. Withering away without much fuss, they are marked for disposal and gobbled up by nearby white blood cells. When you think about it, this process is critical for our bodies to maintain just the right number of cells that they need. Since some 10 billion new cells are produced every day—in places such as the lining of the gut and the surface of the skin, and especially in the bone marrow, where new blood and immune cells are produced—the body has to balance this by making sure that 10 billion other cells quietly disappear.

This targeted self-destruction, also called programmed cell death, is a natural process that makes way for the new and healthy just as a brush fire clears a forest of dead wood to make room for new growth. In the development of the embryo and fetus, programmed cell death prunes unwanted cells to sculpt the developing form, and in the young child's brain, nerve cells that make no important connections fade away.

Suicide genes lie dormant in all our cells, waiting until they get a fateful signal to trigger apoptosis. Old or decrepit cells, and ones containing damaged DNA or deformed chromosomes, essentially volunteer themselves for suicide. When the system is working, apoptosis eliminates rogue cancer cells long before they have a chance to form a tumor mass.

But again, cancer cells can evolve ways to outwit this bodily defense. Blocking apoptosis is an essential prelude to the immortality quest. That this is critical to cancer development was discovered in 1988 when scientist David Vaux and his laboratory found a gene (named bcl-2) that blocks programmed suicide in one form of lymphoma. A few years later the very same anti-suicide gene was discovered in other tumor types, including colon and prostate. As we'll see later, knocking out the protein that keeps cancer cells from taking the poison pill is a logical target for cancer treatment.

The formation of so-called stress proteins is another way injured cells avoid self-destruction. These proteins, also known as heat shock proteins (HSP), make cells resilient to damage, particularly that caused by environmental stress such as high temperatures (hence the name), low oxygen, or toxins, including chemotherapy or radiation. Cancer learns how to become more resilient to therapy by churning out abnormally high levels of these protective proteins. Scientists are at work to see if they can target and reduce the high levels of HSP of certain tumors as a way of making them more susceptible to therapy.

Whether it is the raging cancer cell or the human in search of an earthly everlasting life, the biological paradox is that immortality realized is by necessity lethal. Lethal to neighboring mortal cells, as cancer cells on a god-quest consume the resources destined for others and crowd out essential worker cells. And ultimately lethal to the cancer itself. Selfishly consuming so much energy to sustain its own perpetual life, cancer ultimately drains the life from the very body it is dependent upon for survival. As is so often the case with hubris and narcissism, cancer's avarice leads inexorably to its demise— along with the body that once sustained it. The goal, of course, is to tame cancer's rampant growth before its greed can kill.

Genes That Spur Perpetual Growth

Turning on the telomerase gene and turning off the suicide gene are both necessary for cancer to progress, but they are by no means sufficient. An assortment of other genes also must act up in order to drive a cell to grow relentlessly or to develop the power to take on—and take over—the universe of healthy cells within the body. It is this extensive assortment of abnormal genes that gives each cancer its own distinctive gene profile.

Bit by bit we have learned of categories and hierarchies of the genes that are part of cancerous transformation. Among the first of these oncogenes was a gene called *src*, discovered in the early 1970s by J. Michael Bishop and Harold Varmus, who studied it in birds. If the gene's activity was blocked, tumors did not develop. It was hoped that cancer's long-hidden secret had finally been revealed—the genetic trigger that makes good cells go bad or a quiet cell start to grow uncontrollably.

But such a simple notion, or a single molecule, could not capture the essence of cancer's cunning. In 1982, molecular biologist Robert Weinberg of the Whitehead Institute at MIT discovered the first human oncogene that stimulates unrestrained cell growth. Since then scientists have found numerous other cancer-related genes and identified their proteins, teaching us that cancer commands its own genome, carrying on almost as a novel species, an alien parasitic lifeform.

Oncogenes

Cell division normally begins with the tightly coiled DNA opening up to start copying itself in response to signals triggered from outside the cell. The messages are carried along from the cell surface to its nucleus by a series of proteins that make up growth-signaling pathways. These signaling pathways resemble bucket brigades as they carry chemical messages from one activated protein (coded from one gene) to the next in relay. The human genome is loaded with genes that make up these metabolic routes, and when the genes start barking out inappropriate orders to divide in an uncontrolled way, any one of them can become an oncogene. Oncogenes behave this way either because they are slightly twisted versions of normal genes that get stuck in the "on" position due to a mutation, or because they have been mistakenly copied into the genome too many times and compulsively overproduce growth signals.

Oncogenes can form at many points along this relay: growth factors outside the cell, specific growth receptors on the cell membrane that these factors lock onto, other proteins inside the cell that pick up signals from receptors and relay them to the cell nucleus, and ones that interact directly with the DNA to trigger or sustain the cell division process.

Identifying specific oncogenes sheds light on the behavior of individual tumors. Researchers have discovered many examples, with more to come. One called *erb* codes for the epidermal growth factor receptor, or EGFR. This gene lives on the short arm of chromosome 7, and while it was first identified in normal skin cells, when mutated it plays a role in the development of malignant skin cancers as well as many other malignancies, including leukemia and cancers of the lungs, ovaries, colon, head, neck, and brain. EGFR falls into a class of proteins called tyrosine kinases that are frequent oncogenic catalysts.

Another tyrosine kinase oncogene, *HER2/neu*, is a growth factor receptor gene that is amplified in some breast cancers to produce excess amounts of the HER2 receptor protein. As I will discuss in Chapter 10, the presence of the gene in a tumor indicates more aggressive behavior, and that has led to an entirely new therapy using the drug Herceptin (trastuzumab). The drug benefits women with the gene and offers no value to those without it. If you ever wondered why it was important to know about the ways in which any given cell becomes a cancer, the translation of that knowledge into targeted treatment says it all.

Occurring farther along the growth signaling chain inside the cell is another protein (also a tyrosine kinase) known as BCR-ABL. This is an oncogenic protein central to the development of chronic myelocytic leukemia; the protein is a product of the Philadelphia chromosome mentioned in Chapter 3. (Again, knowing this led to the design of the drug Gleevec.) Another growth driver is a gene called *myc*. It's normally located on the long arm of chromosome 8. In one form of childhood lymphoma, however, this gene is broken and swapped into other chromosomes (2, 12, and 22). This oncogene is also multiplied many times over in some lung and breast cancers, and frequently shows up in tumors as they become more aggressive in their growth and spread.

Some oncogenes do more than stimulate cell growth. They can instead serve as the protectors of cells that are growing inappropriately by interfering with the internal suicide mechanism (apoptosis) that would ordinarily take out a renegade cell. An important onco-gene called *bcl-1* is one such example, found in B-cell lymphoma and other cancers.

All told, the human genome contains more than a hundred oncogenes that work together in different ways. Depending on the mix of these oncogenes, distinct cancer genomes program the de-ranged metabolism that underlies specific tumor types. A major goal of those who are searching for new cancer therapies is to map the many and varied proteins that make up the deranged metabolic net-works for any given malignancy. Studying those maps, just as ex-plorers would assess new terrain, scientists can identify the key proteins that both trigger and sustain cancer. That information, in turn, becomes the blueprint for revolutionary therapies, which I will discuss further in Part Four.

In the most general of terms, traditional therapy (radiation or chemotherapy) goes for the misbehaving DNA, trying to block it from copying itself, and damaging it to the point of self-destruction. But therapy informed by the genetic and metabolic characteristics of a specific tumor can augment the direct DNA attack, zooming in with designer chemicals to block precisely the cancer-stimulating proteins on the surface or inside the cancer cell. The two ap-proaches complement each other.

Suppressor Genes

Our genome does not sit idle as cancer genes run wild. Built into our genetic code are more than thirty tumor suppressor genes, good guys that specifically search for and rein in recklessly multiplying cells. They counter tumor growth, and if need be destroy a hope-lessly misbehaving cell by triggering apoptosis. This built-in genetic defense squad guards the genome and counters the disruptive growth driven by oncogenes.

When we talk about inheriting a susceptibility to cancer, we usually mean that one of a pair of suppressor genes is abnormal at birth. Remember, genes come in pairs, one from each parent. And when cancer susceptibility is inherited from one parent through genes in the sperm or egg—that is, the germ line—the error shows up in every cell in the body, not just in the tumor itself. Geneticists can figure out whether an abnormal suppressor gene in any given cancer genome is inherited from parents or acquired through living by searching for the damaged gene in other tissues of the body, such as the white blood cells or cells that line the inside of the mouth. If one of a pair of suppressor genes is lost there, too, that particular genetic error has been inherited. This also means all relatives sharing that gene deficiency are prone to cancer as well—but not destined to get it.

Because only one-half of a suppressor gene pair needs to be healthy in order to pump out its protective protein, inheriting a damaged gene from one parent doesn't mean you will necessarily get cancer. For the suppressor function to be completely lost, both genes in the pair must be inactivated. Thus, a damaged suppressor gene doesn't become a problem until, in the course of living, the second of the gene pair gets knocked out by mutation—and then the loss of tumor suppression capacity enables the cancer-promoting genes to run wild. In cases where both suppressor genes are normal at birth, the loss of both copies of a suppressor-gene pair can develop over time.

Suppressor genes work in different ways in their effort to produce proteins that keep cells from transforming into cancer. Some literally scan the genome right after the chromosomes are copied, but before the cells split in two. They are the cell's spell checkers, busily proofreading the genome and correcting any mistakes. Losing these editing programs makes cells rapid mutators and allows for gene errors to pile up.

Like oncogenes, tumor suppressor genes take many forms. Hereditary colon cancer involves a suppressor gene mutation that knocks out the *APC* (adenomatosis polyposis coli) gene, which serves as a master switch to put the skids on cell growth. A suppressor gene that is lost in another form of inherited colon cancer, hereditary nonpolyposis colorectal cancer (HNPCC), makes cells less able to repair damaged DNA segments. Defects in the cancer-suppressor genes *BRCA1* and *BRCA2* (located on chromosomes 17 and 13, respectively) figure prominently in hereditary breast cancer. Since these inherited breast cancer genes are present in all cells in the body, it is no surprise that they also increase the risk of cancer in other tissues such as the ovary, prostate, and colon.

The "avenging angel," formally known as *p53* and residing on the short arm of chromosome 17, is one of the foremost cancer suppressor genes—so important that it appeared on the cover of *Science* magazine in 1993 with the designation "Molecule of the Year." This particular gene features prominently in many different cancers, being inactivated or totally lost in more than half of all malignancies. It is also one of the cancer mutations frequently passed on through families. This suppressor gene has many functions. It slows down cell growth to allow time for natural repair mechanisms to work; it also triggers a suicide gene when damage to the chromosome is too extensive to be repaired. But *p53*'s power is also its fatal weakness; if this protector gene itself is damaged, the cell is left largely defenseless against cancerous transformations. Indeed, the loss of *p53* function late in the course of cancer progression often marks a shift to a more aggressive stage in tumor behavior, and frequently a resistance to drug or radiation treatments that may have worked before—perhaps because the therapy had been tricking the gene into forcing the cancerous cell to self-destruct. One of the goals of modern cancer therapy is to learn these cancer tricks and find a way to help the body recover its own healing powers to counter them.

CHAPTER 5

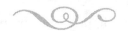

Cancer on the March

AFTER HEARING OF A malignant tumor, invariably the next question that comes to a person's mind is "Has it spread?" That is the right question to ask, not only for assessing our personal outcome, but also for understanding how cancer works and how it can be stopped.

If all that malignant cells could do was to clone themselves indefinitely, they would be shut down. They would use up all of their food, be starved of oxygen, or simply run out of room to grow. But as part of their mission to live forever, malignant cells acquire other critical talents. They rely on both demolition and construction skills to achieve their ends—in this case, displacing productive cells with tumors. They also devise transport systems to carry malignant cells from their primary source out to colonize once-pristine territory in distant organs.

Local Invasion

Under normal circumstances, physical space constraints—bumping up against a neighbor—put a brake on excessive cell growth. But cancers become adept at ignoring biological fences and boundaries. The invasive tentacles of cancer are visible to the naked eye—a characteristic that earned cancer its name more than 3,000 years ago. The Greek physician Hippocrates observed that many tumors—breast, stomach, skin—shared a common feature of irregular margins, with numerous legs sprouting into surrounding areas. He linked these seemingly different conditions with a common name: *karkinos*, Greek for "crab." It is the shorter Latin word for "crab," *cancer*—used by Celsus and another famous Roman physician of old, Galen—that has lasted to this day. In modern terms, Hippocrates's observation surely would be worthy of a Nobel Prize. He keyed in on a cancer trait that, regardless of tumor type, is still used by pathologists to determine whether a tumor shows signs of invasion and therefore malignancy.

A cluster of microscopically cancerous cells that have not invaded surrounding tissue is sometimes designated as pre-malignant, or in-situ cancer, which typically means that the cancer has not yet extended beyond surface cells and broken through the fibrous barriers that separate layers of different tissue from each other. For example, in-situ cancer of the colon means that the superficial lining cells of the gut have been affected, but not those deeper in the gut wall. These are the earliest of cancers, a few cells gone wrong.

As mentioned earlier, oncologists routinely use a system that assigns solid tumors to different grades and stages. Grade is the microscopic description of how differently cells look from the normal cells when studied under the microscope, with lower grades indicating the tumor cells that look closest to normal. Stage marks the progression of cancer in the body: whether it's invaded, how much so, and if it's spread to distant sites. Higher stages are the more advanced.

This established classification system is currently used to compare tumors and guide therapy. It is almost sure to be rewritten in the future as we more precisely characterize a tumor's molecular signature based upon the nature of the genes and proteins that explain and often predict the behavior of individual cancers, including their proneness to spread.

⟿ CLASSIFYING CANCER ⟿

This general classification system creates a common language to define the nature and extent of any given cancer in comparison with other tumors, and is used to assess prognosis, guide treatment, and perform clinical studies and trials. It also informs four questions patients should ask their doctor.

Cell type: What's the cell and tissue of origin?

There are several broad groupings of tumors based on the primary site of development.

~ *Carcinomas involve the coating or lining of organ cavities or ducts. Included are the most common cancers of lung, breast, prostate, colon, and skin. Added descriptors such as* small cell, squamous, *or* adeno-, *further distinguish tissue of origin.*

~ *Sarcomas develop in the body's connective tissue, such as bone and muscle.*

~ *Liquid cancers, including leukemia and lymphomas, originate in cells of the bone marrow or lymph nodes.*

~ *Cancers of the brain and spinal cord arise in stem cells of the nervous system.*

Grade: How abnormal are the cells under the microscope?

Grades are assigned based on the cells' appearance under the microscope, and depend on how much they deviate from normal. Higher grades are more malignant, correlating with more aggressive growth.

~ *Grade I: Cells fairly similar to normal healthy cells of origin; they are "well-differentiated."*
~ *Grade II: Abnormal cell structure and tissue patterns*
~ *Grade III: More marked variation from the normal*
~ *Grade IV: Bizarre, primitive, and poorly differentiated cells*

Stage: How far has the cancer spread?

Stage is based on the extent to which the cancer has spread beyond its primary site of origin; higher stages indicate greater spread. The following apply to solid cancers:
~ *Stage 0 (in-situ): Noninvasive, doesn't extend beyond the superficial cell layer*
~ *Stage I: Penetrates the superficial cell layer to invade the primary organ*
~ *Stage II: Local spread, sometimes to nearby lymph nodes*
~ *Stage III: More severe local and regional spread with lymph node involvement*
~ *Stage IV: Metastasis to distant sites, most often liver, bone, brain, or lungs*

Molecular signature: Are there specific genes that further characterize and help us understand an individual tumor's behavior?

Numerous genes go astray in any given cancer, and when identified can further aid in the classification of cancers of similar type, grade, and stage. Already used in some cases to assess prognosis and target therapy, but still a work in progress.
~ *Oncogenes and their proteins that drive growth*
~ *Lost suppressor genes/proteins that keep malignant cells from suicide*
~ *Genes/proteins that enable cancers' distant spread*
~ *Overall multi-gene or chromosome patterns that indicate prognosis*

In-situ Cancer

Identifying in-situ or stage 0 cancer takes proactive screening. As only a microscopic clump of errant cells, they have not yet formed a tumor that can be felt or seen, and they produce none of the symptoms typical of cancer, such as bleeding or pain. Two of the most common forms of in-situ cancer are those detected in the cervix and the breast, but in-situ disease is also detectable in the bladder, prostate, and colon.

Such early cancer identification can be a blessing, but it also presents a challenge in terms of just when and how to act on those early cancer clusters. (See Part Four.) Indeed, it is not uniformly agreed that these isolated, noninvasive cancer cells found in a milk duct, floating in a urine specimen, or noted in a prostate biopsy will always become invasive cancer, and if so, over what stretch of time. Do these malignant cells have the full suite of deadly skills needed to initiate an attack on the body? We are not sure—but there is little doubt that at least in a meaningful number of cases, in-situ cancers become invasive.

The dilemma for patients and doctors is how to decide what to do when faced with a lack of information on what the cells will do in the years ahead. There is no simple guideline here. The grade of the cancer cells—how hostile or benign they look under the microscope—is one consideration to prompt a more or less aggressive approach. In time, a combination of grade along with the genetic properties of the cancerous cells will help inform these decisions.

Invasive Cancer

Invasive cancer starts out small and advances through stages, even if its particular path and schedule are not always predictable. The onset of invasion, the first stage, is what prompts oncologists to label a tumor malignant. In stage I, invasive cancer advances within its home tissue. When the cancer moves into nearby vessels or lymph nodes, it's characterized as stage II or III, depending on how widespread it is. In the most advanced stage, IV, the tumor has scattered its malignant seeds to distant parts of the body. This quality of invasion represents an extraordinary feat on the part of cancer cells, and it is very much at odds with a body full of organs and systems that are trained to cooperate yet honor each other's territory.

To turn the stage 0 cancer into an invader requires a major construction job. And the process of preparing the soil, building roads, and linking up an energy supply once again takes full advantage of the body's existing resources and talents for this kind of work—expertise already programmed into the cells' genetic code. These include a number of factors and processes listed below.

The Matrix

Matrix became a popular word when its namesake movie offered up evocative images of good and evil having it out in a jelly-filled space created by powerful computers. Imagine a matrix at the cellular level: a place where cells are both captive and connected to each other in a three-dimensional space. Cancer cells with a bent toward invasion need a conduit through this matrix, and one that is a welcoming place for them to take root. The biological matrix that surrounds and supports cells in the tissues and organs of the body is something that is only recently getting attention for its role in the march of cancer.

The extracellular space is packed with an amorphous gel of carbohydrates and proteins, reinforced by strings of the tough, elastic connective protein, collagen. Cells organize into tissues by anchoring themselves to the 3-D collagen web of the matrix. Perfused with nutrient-filled plasma, the matrix provides passage to a veritable soup of chemicals and cells that seep in from the bloodstream and lymphatic system, including immune-reactive white blood cells. At the same time, it acts as the communications infrastructure for ongoing interactions between the traveling cells and the local community of cells that are bound in place.

Cancer takes advantage of the matrix in every way it can to edge out these normal cells and usurp their domain. Sometimes the matrix is resistant to the cancer cells as they try to drill through the collagen web, providing a first line of defense against the cancer attack. In other cases, the surrounding microenvironment not only is a pushover for the bad guys but also turns traitor, becoming complicit in the invasion. Certain tumors secrete a family of enzymes that work like meat tenderizer, helping the cancer cells break away from their matrix restraints and tunnel through the surrounding space, dissolving whatever lies in their path. The extracellular space also has a mix of proteins that can counter these destructive enzymes, making the soil more or less receptive to cancer's march. Researchers are only beginning to understand the back-and-forth battles that are silently waged in this microscopic world.

Angiogenesis

Multiplying cells need a good blood supply. Otherwise, they wither up and die for want of oxygen and nutrients, and choke on an excess of carbon dioxide and the other waste products of normal metabolism. Angiogenesis, the growth of new blood vessels, is a fundamental process in the normal development of a growing child and in wound healing and repair. It is also vital to cancer growth, as tumor cells co-opt the natural mechanisms of angiogenesis to divert blood flow for their own growth. These new blood vessels are so important to cancer's progress that an entire generation of scientists, led by the Harvard researcher Judah Folkman, has been searching for ways to block angiogenesis. (More on this in Part Four.)

As Folkman has been preaching for years—memorably to my second-year class at Harvard Medical School when he was a young professor there—it's simple logic: if cancer cells can't hijack angiogenesis to set up a new blood supply, the cancer mass would not be able to grow much larger than the size of a pencil point. We know now that cancer cells do indeed secrete chemicals that induce the formation of their own network of blood vessels. Vascular endothelial growth factor (VEGF) is an important ingredient for all blood vessel development, and the ingenious cancer cells take over the controls for the normal gene that makes this protein whenever they need it to boost their own blood supply. The new vessels tap into the surrounding tissues' vascular tree, and thus siphon off blood meant for the healthy neighbors.

The newly sprouted blood vessels are normal in cellular structure, but their organizational pattern reflects the chaotic and undisciplined cell designs of the tumor. Normally, blood vessel networks spread out in an open branching pattern much like a well-maintained shade tree. Tumor networks usually look more like the branches in a bird's nest—densely packed and heavily intertwined. The new vessels are also leakier than established ones, causing them to bleed more easily. That's why blood in the sputum, stool, or urine can be the first sign of a hidden cancer.

Inflammation

Another of the body's maintenance tools that is railroaded into cancer construction duty is inflammation. Ordinarily this core function helps to defend against invading pathogens, and helps the body repair wounds and react to injury. It's suspected that in some cases the inflammatory process can wipe out even advanced tumors through a targeted immunological attack. But more routinely, in cancer's world the inflammatory process is commandeered to do just the opposite: to promote invasion and tumor spread.

Inflammation is an experience known to everyone—a searing toothache, a sprained ankle, a skinned knee, or a bad head cold. The red-hot, often painful swelling in an area of injury (the *rubor, calor,* and *dolor* of Celsus) reflects the surge of fluid-borne white blood cells and chemicals that rush to the site, where they loosen up the matrix and encourage cell growth. This stimulates blood vessels to sprout and helps to clear out dead cells, while laying down loose scar tissue to replace them.

In the mid-nineteenth century, the famous German pathologist

Rudolf Virchow proposed that chronic inflammation might actually be the cause of cancer, since he repeatedly observed the many white blood cells that infiltrated the tumors he studied under the microscope. Virchow's theory was not widely accepted at the time, largely because it could not be proven. Inflammatory cells might arrive after the fact; they might be there to help or to hurt, or perhaps just be curious bystanders. We now have good evidence that these special forces of the immune system can actually be summoned by the expanding tumor cells and bamboozled into betraying the very body they were meant to protect.

As part of their selectively activated genome, cancer cells produce inflammation-promoting chemicals called cytokines and chemokines. These are immunological distress signals, and it is the white blood cells, summoned from near and far, that rush in to save the day. With them comes a brew of chemicals that soaks the hot tumor bed in angiogenic factors that induce blood vessel formation, and other compounds that soften up the tissue scaffold, inadvertently opening up more space for the tumor mass to expand.

The white blood cells should be working hard to quell the cancerous mutiny, gobbling up every cancer cell they encounter. But the rogue cells manage to reap the benefits of inflammation while avoiding the dangers. Inflammation is a process best suited to fighting alien invaders, such as infectious bacteria. Cancer cells are more like homegrown insurgents—well versed in the local environment and able to pass for peaceable noncombatants. Coating their outer surface with molecules that help them blend in with the surrounding healthy cells, cancer cells manage to slip through the white blood cells' dragnet. Yes, as Virchow noted long ago, inflammatory cells infiltrate virtually all full-blown tumors, but for the most part they are there to help the tumor—not the patient struggling to fend off the cancer.

Metastatic Cancer

Not content with local domination, almost all cancers are colonial-
ists, spreading into distant organs by a process known as metastasis.
Cancer that has metastasized is cancer in its most advanced stage,
where organs far from the primary site of the tumor are invaded and
colonized in turn. The same processes that enable cancer to spread
its tentacles out locally are used, only more so, to take cancer into
the next stage of severity. To spread distantly, cancer cells must master the ability to set off and travel to outlying territories, establish a
beachhead, and then build an outpost where they can thrive in alien
tissues and organs composed of cells of a completely different type.
But not all cancer cells are equal in their power or intent to metastasize; these qualities, too, depend on their specific genetic profiles,
and on the complex web of proteins that enable the aggressive behavior.

One major gene related to the metastatic process is the suppressor gene *NM23*, first identified more than a decade ago in advanced
malignant melanoma. This has been called a border guard gene,
tasked with keeping cells from taking up residency in territories that
are not their own. During early pregnancy, for example, the placenta pumps out the *NM23* gene's protein in quantity, keeping the
growing stem cells of the early embryo and fetus, some of which
wend their way into the mother's bloodstream, from taking up residence in places outside the womb. *NM23* is a master gene that controls a series of others; when it is silenced, as it is in some melanomas
as well as in cancer of the esophagus, pancreas, bladder, and head
and neck, it aids and abets malignant cells as they build their outpost
in foreign territory.

Motility

Like most territorial invaders, cancer cells are restless. Normally,
cells are firmly embedded in the extracellular scaffold that makes up
solid organs; most are homebodies and stay in place for their life-

time. In contrast, cancer cells adhere only loosely to neighboring cells and the surrounding matrix, and are prone to breaking free and moving about. As noted earlier, they cut a path for their journey by spewing out enzymes to degrade barriers such as collagen that stand in their way. This is critical for local invasions, but also for much longer journeys. Cancer cells are able to poke through thin-walled blood vessels and lymph channels, gaining access to the body's transportation network—and using it to hasten their deadly spread.

The wanderlust of cancer cells is a property they share with some perfectly normal stem cells. Embryonic stem cells travel throughout the growing embryo in a tightly choreographed ballet of rapid development to form a fetus. Normal adult stem cells are motile, too, roaming about in their own specialized organs, and on occasion moving off to distant sites as well, if properly signaled to do so. For example, adult stem cells from the bone marrow have been shown to migrate to the brain, where they apparently become resident neurons in brain tissue. Not surprisingly, this process of motility and migration is also under tight genetic control.

Passage

Cancer cells spread throughout the body by hitching a ride through blood vessels and lymphatic ducts. When cancer transits in the lymph system, it leaves its footprints in the lymphatic way stations, the lymph nodes. This is why analysis of nearby lymph nodes removed at surgery has become a standard way of assessing whether a primary tumor has spread beyond its organ of origin. The general formula is that the larger the number of local lymph nodes that show signs of cancer's passage, the more advanced the spread.

When the invading cells travel instead through blood vessels and into the small capillaries that nourish tissues, they use their drilling skills to burrow back out through the vessel walls, gaining access to the tissue and a possible new home.

Cell-sorting technology now exists that is able to measure minute numbers of tumor cells circulating in the blood. In cancer patients, those numbers are in the range of just one to ten cells per regular-sized vial of blood (a vial is about 7 cc and contains hundreds of millions of cells). Not surprisingly, the higher the number of circulating cancer cells, the greater the tumor load in the body. But cancer cells are not the only stowaways that find their way into the bloodstream, and their presence in the blood does not per se mean the tumor has metastasized. Benign tumors also shed cells into the blood (though at a lower rate than malignant growths), and they do not take up residence or replicate elsewhere in the body to form new tumors. *Benign* is also the word for the stem cells produced by a fetus during pregnancy that can circulate in the mother's bloodstream for years—perhaps even helping her out with needed organ repairs. The point is that the more primitive cells—the normal cells that make up growing embryos, the adult stem cells trying to repair organ damage, and the deranged cancer cells that make up tumors— are skilled travelers and survive in transport.

Magnetism

Securing safe passage is still not enough to ensure a successful invasion, however. There must also be some beacon that draws the circulating cells to a home that will receive them. Most cancer cells that float in the body's circulatory system either don't survive the journey or are unable to take root in distant organs once they get there. That's where magnetism comes in.

Certain organs are more likely to be colonized by cancer than others. The liver, lungs, bones, and brain are the organs most vulnerable to metastases; other organs, such as the heart and the skin, are more resistant. What is gradually becoming clear is that cancer cells target those distant organs that inadvertently put out a welcome mat. For a metastatic cluster of cells to take hold, the new organ of residence must provide fertile ground for their growth, and in turn, the cancer cell must disguise itself as an acceptable guest. A kind of magnetic attraction makes this possible. One example of such mutual affinity is seen in the particularly aggressive form of breast can-ccr that carries the *HER2/neu* gene. These cancer cells wrap their wolf nature in sheep's clothing, coating their outer surface with the HER2 receptor protein, which makes the cell look just like a white blood cell. When distant sites in distress put out a call for white blood cells as part of an inflammatory response, it is the HER2-bearing cancer cells that respond. It's like calling the police to the scene of a mugging and having robbers disguised as cops arrive instead.

Remission of Cancer

The range of tricks, subterfuge, and brute force available to cancer cells can seem at first overwhelming. Indeed, it often is to our bodies when we are attacked from within, and to our minds when we try to work out all the details of a stunningly complex set of diseases. But we know—as with Peregrine Laziosi, who spontaneously recovered from his cancer—that even the most advanced and aggressive of cancers, already infiltrating organs throughout the body, can mysteriously disappear. For reasons we don't yet understand, the encroaching force falters almost at the moment of triumph—like an invading navy suddenly wiped out by a hurricane—and the vulnerable shores are spared. Remarkably, a remission, whether due to medical therapy or occurring spontaneously, seems to be a gentle process, a quiet apoptosis, like leaves falling off a tree in a mild breeze. But how does this happen? Answering that question may be the single most important piece of cancer science that has yet to be done.

Spontaneous remissions are still medical marvels. They have been documented in the mainstream medical literature for more than a century. Inexplicably, these remissions have included the most advanced tumors, and tumors of all kinds, including leukemia, renal cell cancer, malignant melanoma, and cancers of the lung, liver, and breast. Some scientists remain skeptical, but for others these strange events have spawned several lines of medical research.

Some reports have linked spontaneous remissions to prior bouts of high fever or raging infection, suggesting that fever itself might in some cases destroy the bad cells. Or it may be that the immune system, sufficiently mobilized to combat a serious infection, can at the same time knock out an invading tumor. There are researchers who theorize that the human will and psyche may be playing a role as well.

What most of us will experience are remissions due to therapy. Enduring remissions are called cures. Their beauty is that, for the most part, they are the result of a fundamental understanding of the nature of cancer. One thing is for sure: the more we learn about how cancer forms, how it spreads, and where its vulnerabilities lie, the more effective we will be in creating durable remissions, if not certain cures.

The Path Ahead

Cancer has many genomes, and there is no simple path to malignant change, as we once naively hoped. But we can now explain the conundrum that has baffled cancer doctors and their patients for years: that any two given cancers of the same type can look the same yet behave so differently because of dissimilar molecular profiles. We now have the technology to see deeply and decipher much of the behavior of the cancer cell through its many genetic variations and chemical glitches. In doing so, we can start to treat each cancer—and each patient—as an individual with more targeted and personalized care.

This is the big and transforming idea in cancer research today, and it calls for big and transforming science to move it along. It has inspired the Cancer Genome Atlas (TCGA), an NIH program introduced to decode cancer's many molecular blueprints. Under the joint direction of the National Cancer Institute and the National Human Genome Research Institute, this program enlists leading cancer research centers to undertake a three-year pilot to study sequence three cancers. The three to be studied in this first stage are cancers of the lung and ovary, and glioblastoma multiforme, the most common cancer of the brain. If successful, the Atlas will become a decade-long, billion-dollar effort to study 50 of the more than 200 cancers.

The Atlas will be an instruction book about cancers, a modern classification system describing the tapestry of oncogenes, suppressor genes, and other genetic alterations that define any one cancer at different developmental stages, including the proteins they make and the signals they give. With individual cancer genomes fully explored, the Atlas will serve as the foundation for twenty-first-century progress across the cancer field—and offer a blueprint for therapy for each individual patient. It will also lead oncologists to tailored prescriptions for prevention and early diagnosis of cancers based on an individual tumor's distinct signature.

We know how to produce the Atlas quickly and cheaply, but the Atlas is not without its critics. Some warn that cancer biology is still too poorly understood to really interpret the results of an atlas of complex genomic maps—and, representing a "big science" project, there is fear by some scientists that it will take money from other, smaller projects. Those are arguments I've heard before, as they beset the human genome project back in the early 1990s.

Francis Collins, veteran of the Human Genome Project and the head of the National Human Genome Research Institute, has stood tall on the importance of the Atlas. He bemoans the darkness that envelops cancer and limits its research. Collins uses the old analogy of searching for lost keys on a dark street where there's only one lamppost. You search where there's light, and it's only luck if you find the keys there. For cancer, he says, we need "a thousand lampposts to shed light on the darkness of our ignorance." I couldn't agree with him more. The $30 million or so per year allotted for the Atlas pilot project amounts to little more than pencil dust in the overall NIH budget, and one might argue we should set out to sequence far more than three cancers right away. The cancer war will not be won, and the next generation of cancer treatments will not be ready, without knowing the genetic basis of cancers that touch us, one by one.

In this regard, I'd like to invoke another Peregrine: the peregrine falcon. If St. Peregrine represents the hope that cancer, no matter how advanced, can be pushed into a lifelong remission, then the peregrine falcon represents this new science of swift, precise, and targeted cancer therapy—not an evolution but a revolution in how we wage this decades-long war. Known as the fastest animal on the planet, this amazing warrior bird has wandered the skies over every continent for tens of thousands of years. No earthly prey is safe when caught by the falcon's eye, which can lock onto it from great distance. And as this strong and swiftest of creatures zooms in for the deadly strike, it does so without ruffling the surrounds. In short, it is laser-like with few side effects. Targeted, precise, and cleanly lethal, the falcon may be a better metaphor for our coming battles with cancer than is the blockbuster brutality of conventional war.

The genomic revolution offers the vision to decipher cancer's origins, sort out its complex pathways, and target its cells with the precision of a peregrine falcon seeking its prey. That alone creates the imperative for the public to call for a new and accelerated war against cancer, as it did almost four decades ago.

PART THREE

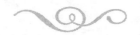

Can We Control Our Fate?

Our remedies oft in ourselves do lie,
which we ascribe to heaven.

—ALL'S WELL THAT ENDS WELL,
WILLIAM SHAKESPEARE

CHAPTER 6

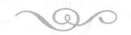

Cancer Risk Factors

WHEN SUDDENLY FACED WITH a diagnosis of cancer, how easy it is to think, *Why me? I did everything right! Or did I?* I tormented myself with such questions early on. After all, cardiologists are big on prevention—the focus on risk factors such as smoking and high cholesterol has paid off in vastly reduced mortality. This mind-set kept me searching my past for what could have possibly turned a few cells sour. Was it a throwback from growing up in an industrial neighborhood, or living over my parents' poorly ventilated perfume factory, which regularly wafted sweet smells up into our apartment? Maybe it was the formalin and other chemicals I inhaled in the pathology labs. Perhaps the X-ray exposure in the catheterization lab did it, or the X-rays scattered from the portable machines that were wheeled around the hospital wards and intensive care units to snap chest films at all times of the day and night. Up close, we always wore lead aprons; should I have had a lead helmet, too? Everything looked suspicious—from microwaves, transmission towers, and cell phones to my penchant for reading whenever I had a free moment. After a while no part of my past life was spared, until I realized how sense-less—though utterly expected—these musings were.

We all want to control our lives and understand what has hap-pened, particularly at a time of illness, when control seems to be slipping away. We all want to know what could have been done dif-ferently so that our children will be spared. But I finally decided I had had enough of these unproductive, depressing thoughts. We do the best we can, and whether we always do it right or not, things happen. All of us facing cancer, including myself, have to come to terms with the reality of random fate.

That does not spare us, however, from understanding the factors that do make one more or less cancer prone. For one thing, avoiding known risk factors can benefit us, whether it is before or after a diag-nosis of cancer. And it helps us move away from random musings to a more concrete sense of just what this disease is about as we under-stand it today. Here, fact is better than fiction.

Cancer comes with being alive, an unfortunate side effect of having cells that renew themselves through the majesty of self-replicating DNA molecules and make the occasional misstep. So cancerous cells will always be with us, popping up amid our healthy cells like an earthquake without a warning. Nonetheless, some can-cers can be prevented outright; most early cancers can be cured; cancer survivors can stay cancer free. Though the science of cancer prevention and early detection is still young, preliminary results show that it applies broadly to many types of cancers—a strong sug-gestion that it can eventually apply to all.

If ever proof were needed that scientific discovery wed to per-sonal action could shift one's medical fortunes, it is provided many times over by the saga of the NIH-supported Framingham Heart Study. Begun in 1948, the research program has been conducting a precise observation of residents of the small town of Framingham,

Massachusetts, for three generations now. The study uncovered risk factors for heart disease that led to the radical notion that the heart attacks then ravaging middle-aged men in most developed countries might be preventable. At first this was a controversial notion, since it was hard to prove for a disease that took decades to develop, but by the time I entered the profession major research studies were under way looking specifically at what could be controlled. Though heart disease was tied to age, being male, and family medical history, other risk factors could be changed by some combination of personal behavior and medical treatment. From that insight, followed up by scrupulous research, preventive cardiology was born.

Since 1970, we have seen a decline in death rates due to heart disease and stroke of greater than 50 percent—compared to a decline in all forms of cancer deaths of about 3 percent. Many of the lifesaving advances in the treatment of heart disease deserve credit, but most experts agree that a good half of the decline in cardiovascular mortality can be attributed to prevention strategies developed in response to the Framingham study. There is no reason that these successes, which have made heart disease a manageable condition for most patients, should be off-limits to those threatened by cancer instead.

I first learned about cancer prevention in medical school from the tales about Sir Percival Pott, the British surgeon who made a crucial discovery in 1775. Physicians had noticed that scrotal cancer developed in chimney sweeps. But it was Sir Percival who linked the cancer to the black coal tar and soot that covered them from head to toe in the course of their daily climbs up and down the chimney flues of London. Furthermore, Sir Percival is credited as one of the first to identify a job-related cancer. His observations came about a decade after another famous British physician, Sir John Hill, identified a hazardous recreational behavior: he linked tobacco snuff with nasal cancer.

Years later it was learned that both of these cancers shared a common cause—the chemical carcinogens found in the brown-black residues of high-temperature burning. One of the best known of these are the benzopyrenes (part of the family of cancer-causing chemicals known as polycyclic aromatic hydrocarbons, or PAHs), which are found in dangerous doses in the tar and soot that clog chimneys and in the dark, sticky residue of tobacco that stains teeth and fingertips. These compounds are also found in trace levels in air polluted by incinerator exhaust and belching smokestacks. They even form on those deliciously char-grilled meats.

Despite the keen observations of the British physicians and subsequent studies on tar, it took centuries for the medical community to get serious about the dangers of tar and tobacco. In 1962, the British Royal College of Physicians came out with a report based on years of research that definitively connected lung cancer with cigarettes, and suggested a link between smoking and heart disease as well. Two years later the U.S. surgeon general Luther Terry issued a similar document warning Americans of the danger of smoking, particularly with regard to lung cancer. Both reports kicked off major public health campaigns (which continue to this day) to rid the population of the cigarette habit. The reports helped redefine the cultural identity of smoking as a scorned rather than respectable social behavior. But they had an even wider impact by establishing the idea that some common cancers resulted from ordinary exposures and personal habits—in other words, that if their risks could be deciphered, their occurrence could be prevented.

The World Around Us

Though cancer stems from the random mutational events that occur as DNA is copying itself, the world around us has a hand in the process. Most of the time, the exposures that assail our cells as they divide arrive inadvertently and unrecognized in the air we breathe and the sunrise that makes us smile; in the stuff we place in our mouths and from the people we love; in the host of invisible rays that zing down from the cosmos above and the ones that rise up from the earth below. These risk factors can be broadly grouped into chemical and biological carcinogens and electromagnetic radiation.

Chemical and Biological Carcinogens

We live immersed in a bath of chemicals both natural and man-made, so it's no surprise that a handful of the thousands we encounter daily pose a cancer threat—such as constituents of tobacco smoke, or asbestos, or certain forms of toxic mold. But in the course of a long life and in the context of a genome that absorbs many hits before it turns bad, pinpointing the exact cause of a cancer is an exceedingly tricky thing to do. We rely therefore on the best solution we have: laboratory tests conducted on animals, mostly rodents, which are exposed to high doses of chemical suspects to see if cancer develops. It's called the Ames test, after Bruce Ames, a molecular biologist and biochemist from the University of California at Berkeley who pioneered not only the test but also our understanding of the mechanisms involved in carcinogenesis.

Carcinogenic chemicals work by messing with the molecules of DNA in our cells. In most instances, Ames points out, the crucial damage is done by that eternal scourge of mortals, the class of highly corrosive oxygen-containing molecules known as free radicals. In excess, free radicals can damage tissue, and have been identified as contributing to chronic degenerative diseases such as atherosclerosis and Alzheimer's, as well as cancer. These molecules develop from our own oxygen-dependent metabolism as well as from external exposures to such elements as sunlight.

As critical as Ames testing has been for identifying carcinogenic compounds, however, Ames himself is one of the strongest critics of those who he believes overinterpret the results of the high-dose rodent test. Humans are not albino rats, and the lab tests typically study chemical doses far beyond any reasonable one-time human exposure. To identify the culprits behind human cancer with certainty, scientists must be able to quantify a person's exposure to the carcinogen over many years, and somehow tie it directly to specific health damage. This requires long-term studies of large groups of people with and without the exposure. Even then it's not so easy: look how long it took us to prove once and for all the dangers of tobacco as a carcinogen.

Consider this fact, for instance: despite the heavy mix of known carcinogens in cigarettes, inhaled in heavy doses for decades, only about 10 percent of smokers get cancer. Most live on into ripe old age cancer free—though often trailing their oxygen tanks as they wheeze with emphysema or bearing a scar from a coronary bypass operation. That most don't get lung cancer points to the variation among people in their biological defenses against carcinogens and their inherent susceptibility to a given cancer. For relatively less toxic carcinogens present in the chemical and biological stew of everyday life that show up in trace levels measured in parts per billion—such as arsenic or pesticide contaminants in drinking water—it is even harder to track and nail down lifetime exposures, to say nothing of eliminating them entirely.

The National Toxicology Program, located on the North Carolina campus of the National Institute of Environmental Health Sciences of the NIH, gathers information on potential carcinogens and conducts tests in their laboratories. Every two years they generate a report on carcinogens for Congress. The list, available at http://ntp-server.niehs.nih.gov, focuses mainly on the chemical carcinogens. Some, such as soot, cigarettes, and sunlight, are immediately recognizable, but many are unfamiliar chemicals with unpronounceable names.

With one look at this long and ever-expanding list it's clear that since the sun began to shine on the planet and fire was tamed for human use, we have lived in a sea of carcinogens, externally exposed or internally consumed. Along the way the survivors, human and animal, evolved numerous protective mechanisms to detoxify, counter, destroy, or neutralize the carcinogenic assault. Plants are a part of this protective system, offering up a rich set of defenses.

These defenses include the antioxidant chemicals naturally produced or those taken in the diet mainly from plants. They function as a kind of antidote that mops up free radicals before they have a chance to inflict their oxidative damage. Individual cells of the body also come equipped with the means to flush out a full range of toxins in search of trouble. The liver is a giant detox factory for bad chemicals that are made by the body or that enter it through what we drink, eat, and inhale. The body also has sensors that trigger the rejection of bad stuff before it is breathed in or digested, which explains our natural aversions to certain smells or tastes, and the protective sneezing, coughing, nausea, and vomiting when toxic substances are taken in. Even the nausea and vomiting triggered by chemotherapy and radiotherapy show the strength of the body's rejection of genotoxins, despite their role in attacking cancer.

Though the term *carcinogen* often brings to mind some of the fouler inventions of industry, tainting our food or drinking water, environmental contaminants are just as apt to occur naturally. Arsenic is found in soil and rocks. Aflatoxin, a ferocious carcinogen of biologic origin, is the toxic product of a mold called *Aspergillus flavus*, which grows on crops in warm, moist climates. Corn, cottonseed, and peanuts are favored for such moldy growth. The dangers of this toxin to both animals and humans were only recognized in the early 1960s; testing has shown that the contaminant has found its way into produce such as peanuts and peanut butter, wheat, tree nuts, and even dairy products when animals have consumed moldy feed. Although FDA regulations consider very low amounts of aflatoxin as unavoidable in certain crops, they place nanogram-level limits on its presence in foodstuffs fed to both humans and animals. Studies in both Africa and China, where toxic levels of this substance more often wend their way into the national diet, link aflatoxin to liver cancer, particularly when combined with ongoing liver injury from viral hepatitis or parasitic liver infection.

In an effort to quantify just how much of the environmental soup of chemicals people actually take into their bodies, the CDC regularly samples blood and urine of a representative group of the civilian population for compounds ranging from pesticides to tobacco smoke, from heavy metals to plant estrogens. The 2005 "National Report on Human Exposure to Environmental Chemicals" brings good news: the levels of carcinogens in our bodies have decreased compared to previous tests. Among nonsmoking adults, the impact of secondhand smoke is on the decline. The chemical marker in the blood that measures exposure to cigarette smoke, a breakdown product of nicotine called cotinine, has fallen by about 75 percent since the prior testing interval of 1988–1991. Similarly, blood levels of three potentially carcinogenic pesticides, which are no longer in use in the United States thanks to the Environmental Protection Agency (EPA), are now undetectable.

What remains a mystery, however, is the biological meaning of exceedingly low levels of carcinogens measured in parts per billion or per trillion. We don't have a way of quantifying cancer risks at such exposure levels or of estimating how any one individual manages these exposures. What's more, it's difficult to assess cause and effect, or to unravel the confounding reality that ordinarily we are exposed to many carcinogens at once, and that they can enhance each other's risk. Though we don't know all the carcinogens in our daily life, we have learned from the more obvious ones. For example, the combination of alcohol plus tobacco results in a greater risk for head and neck cancer than we would expect from just adding together the increased risk of both exposures taken alone. The same is true for the combination of asbestos and tobacco for lung cancer.

This brings to mind the words of Paracelsus, credited as the founder of the field of toxicology, who in 1567 said: "All substances are poisons; there is none which is not a poison. The right dose differentiates a poison and a remedy." Paracelsus recognized that there is a therapeutic, beneficial, or just plain benign range for any substance and a toxic level as well, and it's often difficult to ascertain the difference.

But applying this to our everyday life is especially difficult. Look at our daily consumption of foods. Millions of people, including my own family, have switched to organic foods and nontoxic household products in an attempt to dodge the bullet of cancer, among other ills. But we have no way of really knowing whether these and other seemingly safer products that we place in our grocery carts are worth the extra expense. We have science-based government regulatory agencies that should be helping us here, but many people are less than sanguine about their performance. By the nature of their work, the agencies draw sharp lines defining something as either good or bad for the population as a whole, without helping us quantify the relative risk of the many exposures we face, naturally or from commercial products. What's the relative risk of farm-raised salmon or hormone-fed cows or the chemicals in shampoo? And what is their cumulative effect over time?

Just because something is sold or readily available or even regulated by the government does not mean it's safe. Look at tanning parlors. Common sense would tell you that they are a cancer risk, yet they seem to be everywhere, attracting our young people in droves. And their customers are given little or no information about the radiation dose or its potential harm.

Clearly, each of us has to find a middle ground between ignoring real or potential risks and living in fear. But it will be hard to get there unless the regulatory agencies become more public and consumer friendly—which means, in some cases, less beholden to the industries they regulate. Whether it's the safety or quality of the air we breathe, the water we drink and the food we consume, or the places we go, we are ever dependent on the forces of government to keep us safe. On this score the accountability of our public officials, the transparency of their decision making, and the vigilance of public advocates are paramount.

Radiation

We cannot escape the reach of ionizing radiation, the silent carcinogens that come from the cosmos, the crust of the earth, the soil and water around us, and the practice of diagnostic and therapeutic medicine. There are many types of ionizing radiation, including subatomic particles such as alpha and beta rays, and electromagnetic radiation, especially gamma rays, X-rays, and the most energetic forms of ultraviolet light. They cause their damage by blasting our atoms and molecules into unstable, electrically charged versions of themselves, but the physical makeup and energy levels of these rays determine the risk they pose. Ionizing radiation has been with humanity as long as we've existed, but its discovery and our awareness of its dangers were accidental events, happening not much more than a hundred years ago.

It was 1895 when Wilhelm Röntgen, a German physics professor, discovered the curious power of the electromagnetic rays emanating from his X-ray machine. A published photo of an X-ray of his wife Bertha's hand with her fourth finger encircled by an opaque wedding band spoke a thousand words. With a technology that was painless—and seemed at least initially to be harmless—the X-ray revealed the dark image of her bony skeleton surrounded by grayer shadows of flesh and skin. Like magic, humans could peer into the body of a living person and gaze at internal body parts; overnight this discovery took off as a grand medical advance. In 1901, Röntgen won the Nobel Prize in physics for this feat.

In the United States, Thomas Edison got into the X-ray act by creating a commercially available fluoroscope, capable of giving real-time moving images of the interior of the living body. But the danger of such miracles quickly became apparent. Edison's assistant, Clarence Daly, was regularly exposed to the hazard, and lost both of his arms due to malignant skin ulcerations. Edison abandoned the X-ray work, but Daly eventually died of radiation poisoning in 1904. At about the same time, Pierre and Marie Curie discovered radioactive materials and the element radium, which had its own power to spontaneously emit X-rays. But they, too, learned early on that this material had the frightening ability to burn through flesh. Marie herself developed skin wounds from exposures to vials of radioactive material she carried about in her pocket, and years later died from leukemia—as did her daughter, Irène, who had worked alongside her.

Still, the true perils of this mysterious new physical energy were not fully appreciated for years to come. Even in the mid-twentieth century, facial acne was casually treated with X-rays; only later was this practice linked to thyroid cancer. At about the same time, shoe stores used X-ray machines to see if your shoes fit. And it was well into the 1980s before radiologists and cardiologists began to wear lead thyroid shields to complement their lead aprons during the course of their work in diagnostic catheterization laboratories.

Ionizing radiation is dangerous just because it's ionizing. That means it rams into atoms with enough energy to knock one of their electrons clean out of its orbit circling the atomic nucleus. The result is a particularly nasty ion, or electrically charged atom, with an insatiable greed for the electrons of its neighbor atoms—those DNA-mangling free radicals. Laboratory experiments show that when DNA is bombarded by ionizing radiation, it mutates rapidly and becomes scrambled by breaks, sometimes so badly that the cell is forced to commit suicide. And this, of course, is why radiation is both a cause of and a cure for cancer.

But not all forms of ionizing radiation present the same level of risk to humans; it depends on how easily they can pass through the outer layer of the skin, which is made up of a see-through thin protective armor of compacted dead and dying epidermal cells. Gamma rays, high-energy X-rays, are the most dangerous because they can invisibly, painlessly, and silently move through clothes and skin and penetrate deeply into the body. It takes concrete or lead to block gamma rays—including the type used to produce medical images.

Beta particles, which often travel in nature along with gamma rays, are more ionizing than gamma rays, but generally less dangerous for people. That's because they can't travel far through solid matter—a sheet of aluminum foil is all it takes to stop them cold. Beta particles from radioactive iodine, for example, can be targeted to a specific organ and used in cancer treatment. Brachytherapy delivers short-range radiotherapy with small radioactive seeds, which are implanted in and around the tumor, emitting beta particles or low-energy gamma rays. The seed itself can filter out the higher-energy radiation. This is commonly used for treating prostate cancer and has been shown to cause less radiation damage to nearby tissues, such as the bladder, compared to more traditional external beam treatment.

Alpha particles are yet another matter. Bigger than beta particles, they pack an even more intense and damaging energy wallop, but fortunately they can be blocked by a thin sheet of paper or by the outer layer of our skin. However, it's hard for us earthlings to escape the touch of alpha. The earth itself sends off alpha radiation in the form of the naturally occurring gas, radon. Odorless and tasteless, this vapor seeps out from the small quantities of radioactive uranium found in some soils and rocks, and sometimes inadvertently baked into bricks. Radon gas rises from the crust of the earth, and is found in especially large quantities in volcanic rock, whether it be on a mountaintop or in a valley. It can also seep into groundwater, and from water into the air. But since alpha particles cannot penetrate the skin, radon can do bodily harm only if it is inhaled, bringing it into direct contact with living tissue. It's estimated that inhaled radon is the second most important risk factor for lung cancer, after tobacco.

According to the EPA, radon gas is naturally present in the outdoor air at very low levels. In most areas, this background radon radiation amounts to something less than a tenth of the exposure believed to pose a small increased risk of lung cancer, though that risk is increased in smokers. However, the gas can build up in poorly ventilated spaces such as basements, particularly when there are cracks in the foundation or exposure to soil, as might occur in crawl spaces. Fortunately, we can decrease our exposure with a regular airing out; sealing off obvious entry points such as sumps and crawl spaces also mitigates the risk. But no earth dweller can entirely escape exposure to radon, and since it is invisible, the only way to know of the exposure is to test the air. You can buy reliable home-testing kits or bring in an expert to measure it for you. If the levels are high, they can and should be lowered; think of it as dealing with a damp basement.

But gamma rays remain the biggest concern. About 20 percent of our lifetime exposure to ionizing radiation comes in the form of diagnostic radiology—from the chest film to the CT scan, the dental X-ray to the radioisotope scan. For any one test the exposure may seem minuscule, but the aggregate amount over a lifetime can add up to an important risk factor. Moreover, this is a controllable one, provided you keep track and don't hesitate to have that discussion with your doctor. I will discuss this further in Chapter 8.

The other 80 percent of our lifetime exposure to ionizing radiation is a consequence of natural radiation from the environment. Radiation's cancer-producing potential is directly related to cumulative, lifetime dose. But let's put this in perspective. We measure radiation exposures in units called grays. Lifetime environmental radiation averages about 10 centigrays (a tenth of a gray) or less. Survivors of the atomic bombs that were dropped on Hiroshima and Nagasaki in 1945, or of the Russian nuclear plant explosion in Chernobyl in 1986, faced radiation levels in the range of 100 centigrays all at once. That tenfold increase is associated with about a 50 percent increase in all cancers—particularly leukemia and breast cancer. Thyroid cancer is another risk recently reported in survivors of the Chernobyl disaster who had been under eighteen years of age at the time. That disaster exposed them to radioactive material containing isotopes of iodine and cesium.

For all the human ability to control—and to lose control of— the power of radiation, however, it is nature that must take the blame for most of our radiation-based cancer. There's the earth beneath our feet, but also the sky above our heads. Cosmic radiation from outer space showers us all; those living on mountaintops face more of these rays, as do frequent air travelers, to say nothing of the rare breed that sets up temporary housekeeping on the International Space Station. (One of the greatest barriers to interplanetary space travel is the problem of protecting astronauts from cosmic radiation.) Our planet has its own protective barriers, such as the ozone layer, which affords some degree of cosmic shielding. The thinning of the ozone layer—in part related to our planetary industrial activity—is something that has important medical implications, particularly for our children and their children.

Fear of What We Cannot See: Non-ionizing Radiation

The other major and invisible form of radiation that surrounds us is the non-ionizing type, the kind that does not generate those nasty free radicals. This also radiates from the sun or is produced by earthling innovations: microwaves, radio waves, infrared radiation, and all the other electromagnetic rays we've harnessed to make our cell phones sing, our remote controls zap, and our MRI machines reveal the details of every millimeter of the human body.

Non-ionizing radiation drives our high-technology world. While it might jazz up some molecules, and sometimes heat them up as in microwave ovens, non-ionizing radiation does not change molecular structures as ionizing rays do. Nonetheless, those high-voltage electric lines and blinking cell phone towers are a persistent source of public fear, which at the very least should prompt continued investigation. And however wonderful they may be to our wired planet, I think it's fair to say that we don't know the cumulative effect, if any, of the many Wi-Fi zones we walk through every day.

As it stands, ultraviolet light from the sun is the only form of non-ionizing radiation that is linked with certainty to malignancies, and that seems to be limited to cancer of the skin. Other forms of non-ionizing radiation have not been shown to be carcinogenic. That goes for the radiation from cell phones, which surrounds us with such growing intensity these days. Several studies have looked for connections between cell phone use and cancer, including brain tumors, but so far none have been uncovered.

The World Within Us: Age and DNA

In part because of external exposure and in part because of growing old itself, cancer is a disease that comes with age. Fully 80 percent of tumors show up in those over the age of fifty. Even if predisposition comes at birth, as with certain genetic susceptibilities, it takes decades for the multiple genetic hits to accumulate and achieve malignant transformation. But cancer prevention is another matter—while it's never too late to start protecting yourself, cancer has a long and un-predictable lead time, and prevention should start with the very young, the earlier the better. For example, teen exposure to blistering sunburns is a risk factor for malignant melanoma in later years. The teen years are also the most dangerous time to take up smoking: com-pared to those who start a decade later, teens who begin smoking in-crease their chances of getting lung cancer. Radiation to the chest is associated with increased risk of breast cancer, but if the exposure is during adolescence (for example, when young girls receive breast ra-diation for Hodgkin's disease), that risk is greatly enhanced. On the other hand, if a woman has her first child after the age of thirty-five, she has a 50 percent greater chance of getting breast cancer compared to women who have their first baby under the age of twenty. This does not mean women should start having babies in their teens, but we should all be aware of the many age-related aspects of cancer risk. Knowing about one's youthful exposures in particular is an important part of constructing a lifelong cancer risk profile.

As important as environmental exposures are, it's also important to remember that heredity accounts for 5 to 10 percent of the risk for most common cancers. Even before we could identify specific genes or gene patterns to explain this, it was known that some families were cancer prone. A family tree in which prostate, breast, colon, or ovarian cancer or malignant melanoma has occurred in first-degree relatives (a parent, sibling, or child) signals a two to three times greater chance of getting one of these cancers compared to those without this family history. A smaller hereditary risk is seen with kidney cancer, non-Hodgkin's lymphoma, pancreatic, stomach, and even lung cancer. In contrast, heredity does not seem to play a role in adult leukemia or cancer of the cervix, uterine lining, or bladder.

Inborn genetic problems weigh most heavily with the cancers that each year affect nearly 10,000 children under the age of fifteen—1,600 of whom die. The most common forms of childhood cancers are leukemia and brain tumors, though the genetic alterations underlying these cancers usually come from mutations that occur early in prenatal life—a time of rapid cell division and growth—rather than from genes inherited from parents. Childhood cancers have been tied to high levels of radiation exposure, and in some recent studies to a deficiency of folate in the mother's pre-pregnancy diet, a deficiency that has been tied to broken chromosomes. Drawing on the analogy to heart disease, childhood cancer is more like congenital heart disease, which is due to developmental error, whereas adult cancer is more like degenerative atherosclerotic changes that occur in coronary arteries and cause heart attacks later in life.

When common cancers such as those of the colon or breast occur in younger people—between the ages of twenty and fifty—there is a greater likelihood of a predisposing genetic susceptibility. As mentioned, the mutated genes that run in families, *BRCA1* and *BRCA2*, are best known for breast cancer that hits women in their thirties and forties, but they are also associated with ovarian, prostate, and colon cancer. Keeping track of relatives who developed cancer, and at what ages, should be part of your own personal medical history. You can't change your heredity or your genes, but you can recognize where the threats lie and be doubly motivated to modify the other risks that are under your control.

What We Can Avoid

When it comes to cancer, there is plenty that we cannot change, and mostly would not want to change if we could: our parents, our early life exposures, or our age. Nor can we block our exposure to the sun or the cosmos, or to the high-tech world of multimedia marvels. But we are not off the hook. There are several responsible things we can do to ward off some cancer risk. A word of caution: this is not a blame game but rather a strategy for those who wish to know what actions they and their family can responsibly take to decrease their state of cancer proneness. And that goes for cancer survivors, too.

Personality, Stress, and Cancer

In 1959, physiologists Meyer Friedman and Ray Rosenman coined the phrase "type A personality" to describe the uptight, touchy, impatient, competitive, and at times hostile sort prone to high blood pressure and heart attacks. Though this linkage has never been conclusively proven, it ushered in some rather convincing research on the impact of personality on many aspects of health. And no doubt the concept of type As has become well entrenched in popular thinking because it bears at least a grain of truth.

The personality poison that comes up most often for the heart is the hostile, aggressive sort. This is something to be avoided, for one's own heart and everybody else's. As for other elements of type A personalities—striving, pushing for high standards, being impatient for good results, and working hard and intensely—give such people a break. If they can strive with joy, that's a winning formula. If, however, they are full of misery and frustration, they need a dose of type B. That's the mellow, more easygoing type.

Similar attempts to capture the essence of a distinctive cancer-susceptible personality have been made. Some researchers linked breast cancer to the type A personality; that has not stood up. Less well known is the work of the renowned British psychologist Hans Eysenck, who himself died of cancer in 1997. In 1962, he gave cancer a type all of its own, which has been labeled appropriately as C—very different from types A and B. Eysenck characterized the personality of male lung cancer patients as being very nice—a stereotype that might be captured as "You are just *too nice*—that's why you got cancer."

Eysenck's type Cs are appeasers who assert little and repress much. They are self-sacrificing and tend to come across as calm and patient people. But beneath the surface, type Cs teem with discontent. Lydia Temoshok, a psychologist at the University of Maryland, elaborated on such individuals in her book *The Type C Connection*. She notes that they swallow anger, suppress anxiety and emotions, and are entirely *too* calm and pleasant, belying an inner turmoil that can literally suppress the immune system and drive physical illness. Temoshok makes a case for behavior modification as a strategy for cancer prevention. But just as sending type As to yoga class has never proved itself as a way to prevent heart attacks, neither has the type C personality surfaced as a modifiable cancer risk factor. In fact, the evidence for a type C connection with cancer has been sharply challenged by many other studies from all over the world.

With closer scrutiny most evidence suggests that cancer is an equal personality offender. Introverts and extroverts, depressives and hotheads, As, Bs, and Cs are all touched by this disease. In one of the largest studies of its kind, Japanese researchers reported in the *Journal of the National Cancer Institute* in 2003 that when it came to cancer incidence, individual personality just did not matter. A behavioral medicine research team from Tohoku University monitored more than 30,000 people and, using the personality questionnaire developed by Eysenck, separated them into four different categories of temperament: outgoing and agreeable, anxious and emotionally fragile, aggressive and cold, and conformist and deceptive. Cancer affected all groups without distinction, and without significant differences in number or type—though the investigators did find correlations between cancer and family history, tobacco use, and alcohol consumption.

Stress is one dimension of psychology that cuts across all personality types, and there is accumulating evidence that it may be a risk factor for cancer. The relatively new field of psychoneuroimmunology, or PNI, studies the effect of stress on the immune system. Personal experience teaches—and many studies have shown—that stressful life events can become health risks. The stress of caring for a chronically ill family member, losing a spouse, marital strife, social isolation—all of these can depress components of the immune system. Psychologist Jan Kiecolt-Glaser and immunologist Ronald Glaser at Ohio State University see a strong basis for linking psychological stress with certain cancers since chronic stress depresses white cells that fight cancer and can interfere with DNA's ability to repair itself.

While indirect measures, these observations continue to provide enough circumstantial evidence to keep the notion of a stress-cancer link very much alive. It's quite plausible that a depressed immune system with a less robust army of roving white blood cells that specialize in searching out and destroying invaders would increase susceptibility to cancer development, especially when other predisposing conditions exist.

But the question remains: do stress relievers such as social support make a difference when it comes to avoiding or beating cancer? My bet is yes. Having a circle of concern and love around you is medicine. And listen to the heart: there is evidence that people who have major heart attacks fare better if they are married and have strong social networks. When it comes to cancer, it's only a matter of common sense that a constructive attitude and a sturdy immune system are health-promoting, cancer risk or not. The right attitude is at the heart of cancer prevention, for there is no simple pill here. It requires work to modify behavior—to eat healthily, shun cigarettes, limit sun exposure, and stick with a program of regular cancer screening. Perhaps the personality type we should be looking for here is the anti-cancer personality—namely, someone who has the will to learn and take charge of his or her own personal risks.

Smoking

As far as I'm concerned, we cannot hear enough about the dangers of smoking, at least until the last cigarette gets snuffed out. There are few medical facts that have been established more clearly than the link between cancer and smoking. Tobacco smoke distributes hundreds of cancer-producing chemicals to the nose, mouth, throat, and lung, and from there through the blood to other organs of the body. It should be no surprise, then, that lung cancer is not the only smoking-related cancer.

Smoking is also linked to cancers of the mouth and throat, pancreas, stomach, bladder, kidney, colon, cervix, and uterus, and to myelogenous leukemia. This, along with the fatal damage the toxic weed does to the body's blood vessels, heart, and lungs, makes it the terror of all times. Humans were simply not meant to smoke tobacco. Yet with its satisfying blends that stimulate the pleasure-providing nicotine receptors in the brain to the point of addiction, it's a habit that has infected every city and hamlet on the planet. The World Health Organization estimates that 650 million people currently smoke, and half of them will die from the habit.

Here in the United States we have been aggressively pursuing smoke-free initiatives for years. It's been hard going at times, but the work is paying off. Most of us can see the differences in our homes and at work, on airplanes and in public places. Earlier in my career, a large fraction of my medical colleagues were heavy smokers, and medical conferences often took place in smoke-filled rooms. When I think of those times, I can't help but recall the famous Lasker Award–winning Cleveland Clinic cardiologist Mason Sones, who revolutionized care of the heart patient by developing coronary arteriography. But he was also famous for smoking—even lighting up outside the catheterization lab right after performing his meticulous studies of this smoking-provoked disease. Tragically, he died of lung cancer when he was in his early sixties. But most medical docs got religion, and the culture changed almost overnight. Gone were the ashtrays at medical meetings; preaching against cigarettes became medical creed. And with major public health campaigns, the word did get out. There are still many smokers, of course, but precious few who could claim not to know that it is killing them.

In less than a generation, cigarettes have gone from being part of the fabric of daily life, with about 50 percent of American men smoking, to about half that number today. However, women—who rarely smoked (at least in public) before the women's movement of the 1960s—stepped quickly into the breach, despite stacks of surgeon generals' reports. This was one bit of equality we all could have done without—women now rival men in their addiction to this skin-aging, mouth-fouling, heartbreaking pleasure, still deeply rooted in culture and behavior. Our biggest challenge now is to keep our young people from developing the habit in the first place. But with seeming indifference to what we have learned the hard way, they continue to take it up, with girls leading the senseless charge. So here we are, over two hundred years after Sir Percival and Sir John made their discoveries, with tar still reigning as number one among the environmental hazards causing the most cancer deaths in the United States and worldwide. It does not have to be that way.

Sun Exposure

The warm and cheery rays of the sun are deliciously unavoidable: we rely on them for growth, light, heat, happy moods, and good health. But the best of things in excess have risks, and skin cancers are on the rise. Ultraviolet rays, though generally non-ionizing, damage the skin and, based on your skin type, your genetic susceptibility, and how much exposure you've had, are the setup for pre-cancerous conditions such as the rough, red spots called actinic keratosis, and for the cancerous transformation of squamous and basal skin cells. Unlike these slow-growing, localized, and easily treated skin cancers (assuming they're caught early on), the deadly malignant melanoma is less tightly linked to the sun—except for the blistering sunburns experienced early in life. Simple but disciplined measures to shield yourself—and especially your children—with sunscreen, hats, and clothing go a long way to ward off skin cancer. It's also a good idea to see your physician or dermatologist for an annual skin check, or if you ever notice a change in the appearance of a mole. It's not hard to start doing regular checks for the signs of melanoma, which are labeled ABCD to make them easy to remember. Ask your doctor about a mole that is <u>a</u>symmetric, if its <u>b</u>orders are irregular, if it has a <u>c</u>olor that is uneven, or if it is larger than 6 millimeters (about a quarter of an inch) in <u>d</u>iameter. It's important to emphasize here that, just as there's no safe tobacco use, there's also no such thing as a risk-free tan. Tanning beds are an absolute no-no, and absent federal action, several states have very sensibly enacted laws that require teens to obtain parental approval before salon tanning. As for the sun, we need common sense. Like most things, the sun is fine in moderation. A little sun might even protect against many forms of cancer, since the skin makes vitamin D with sun exposure, and vitamin D promotes normal cell development. But to get the benefit, all you need is about ten to fifteen minutes outdoors—not a glowing tan.

STDs and Other Infections

Until recently the notion that pathogens posed cancer risk had no standing; in fact, the idea was laughable. I recall a newspaper clipping taken from a religious magazine that hung on the bulletin board of our med school dormitory. The headline was something to the effect of "Sex Causes Cancer" and described unfortunate women who contracted cancer as a result of their sexual activities. The article was there for amusement; we smart medical students knew well that this was a phony way of trying to curtail the behaviors of those caught up in the sixties' sexual revolution. Perhaps it was. But it turned out to be more right than wrong. Since then we have discovered a host of sexually transmitted human pathogens, some old, some new, that increase risk for specific cancers. And that knowledge has enabled us to tame some of yesterday's most wicked malignancies. This does not mean that cancer can be caught like the flu, but it does mean that certain pathogens are carcinogens that over time contribute to the development of malignancies.

Human viruses pack their own genes and, in the process of infecting human cells, commingle their nucleotides with those of their victims. As viruses penetrate cells, they hijack their cellular machinery and transform them into what they were never intended to be—viral manufacturing plants churning out more virus. In the animal world oncogenic viruses are fairly common—they cause mammary tumors in rodents and leukemia in cats. But viruses are less apt to be cancerous agents in humans, and for most of the twentieth century chemical carcinogens and radiation were considered the dominant environmental risk factors.

One of the first convincing examples of human cancer-producing viruses came in the late 1970s when virologist Robert Gallo discovered a virus related to a rare form of human leukemia and lymphoma called human T-lymphotrophic virus type 1. HTLV-1 zooms in on one form of lymphocyte, the T cell, a critical player in the immune system, and can rewrite part of the cell's genetic code, turning it into a malignant form. HTLV-1 leukemia and lymphoma occur most often in Japan, Africa, South America, and the Caribbean. This virus is transmitted via intimate human contact—sexually, through dirty needles, in blood transfusions, from pregnant mother to the fetus, or via breast milk. Since all blood in the United States is screened for HTLV-1, we have learned that as many as 1 out of 4,000 people in the United States carry the virus, but only occasionally does it induce blood cancer. This means that some unknown co-factors are at work, one likely being a weakened immune system.

A few years later Dr. Gallo and his colleagues at NIH, along with virologist Luc Montaigner and scientists from the Pasteur Institute in Paris, discovered another retrovirus, called the human immunodeficiency virus (HIV), as the cause of AIDS. AIDS patients clearly show a connection between viruses and the immune system. Patients with AIDS can develop a rare cancer called Kaposi's sarcoma that infiltrates the skin; it is tied to a herpes virus. Women with AIDS are susceptible to an aggressive form of cervical cancer.

Another herpes virus, the highly infectious Epstein-Barr virus (which causes the "kissing disease," mononucleosis), can also become a factor in cancer. Spread easily on eating utensils and through coughing, sneezing, or kissing, it manages to infect most of the population by the time they are twenty years of age without producing any identifiable illness. On rare occasions, however, it is associated with lymphoma, nasal cancer, and some cancers of the stomach. Yet another member of the herpes family is the well-known genital herpes, which is a factor in various forms of cancer of the reproductive tract in both men and women. But before you panic, know that these viruses are common in the population and their role as biologic carcinogens in otherwise healthy people is relatively rare. This is particularly so if one compares them to the human papillomavirus.

~Human Papillomavirus (HPV)

If ever there was evidence that a biological carcinogen can cause cancer, and that by knocking out that carcinogen the cancer can be avoided, the human papillomavirus, the prime culprit of cervical cancer, is it. There are numerous strains of the virus, many benign, but a dangerous handful, including strains 16 and 18, turn cells bad. HPV causes warts on the genitals and occasionally in the mouth and larynx. (Women with genital warts can transmit them to their infants' respiratory tract at the time of delivery, and their presence is an indication for a cesarean section.) But chronic infection with HPV can also lead to cervical cancer and other less common cancers of the vulva, vagina, anus, and penis. And some evidence points to links between HPV and cancers of the mouth, tongue, tonsils, and throat.

HPV infects about 40 percent of sexually active women at some point in their lives. For most, it's a short-lived infection beaten down by the body's immune system. But for some 55,000 American women each year, the viral infection lingers and, over the course of anywhere from three to fifteen years, advances to an in-situ cancer of the cervix and subsequent progression to invasive cancer. Worldwide, cervical cancer is diagnosed in 470,000 women and kills half of that number each year.

As with other carcinogens, HPV is more likely to cause cancer when there are other associated factors, including co-infection with multiple strains of this virus or with other sexually transmitted diseases, including herpes, chlamydia, gonorrhea, and syphilis. A particularly aggressive form of cervical cancer occurs in women with AIDS, as HPV takes advantage of their suppressed immune systems. Birth control pills have been linked to an increased risk of cervical cancer, leading some to surmise that the contraceptive hormones may predispose the genital environment to persistent HPV infection, though the pill link might also reflect decreased condom use and reinfection.

In a triumph of basic and applied medical science as it relates to public health, two vaccines, Gardasil and Cervarix, have been developed to immunize against the specific cancer-producing strains of HPV. After a twenty-year targeted research effort, Georgetown University cancer researcher Richard Schlegel and colleagues discovered the vaccine technology and turned it over to a relatively small pharmaceutical company, MedImmune, in Gaithersburg, Maryland, to develop an experimental vaccine for early clinical testing. The work was so promising that it was licensed to two of the world's largest pharmaceutical companies: Merck, which produced Gardasil, and GlaxoSmithKline, which produced Cervarix. With their scientific expertise and market muscle, these companies carried out worldwide clinical studies leading to final FDA approval of Gardasil in 2006; Cervarix is on schedule to follow. These vaccines have been shown to be close to 100 percent effective in creating immunity, and should reduce new cases of cervical cancer by 75 percent or more. Meanwhile, Dr. Schlegel and his team are part of a major international effort funded by the Bill and Melinda Gates Foundation and the NIH to develop a next-generation vaccine, which is less expensive and does not require refrigeration, for use in less developed parts of the world where cervical cancer runs rampant. Researchers are also exploring the use of vaccines in treatment of cervical cancer.

~*Hepatitis Virus*
Chronic infection with either hepatitis virus B or C increases the risk for liver cancer. It's now believed that about 30 percent of all cancers

originating in the liver result from chronic hepatitis, and the figure is higher in less developed parts of the world. Both forms of hepatitis can be transmitted sexually through exchange of bodily fluids, and also by using dirty needles. Until the early 1990s, when all blood products began to be screened for both hepatitis B and C with newly developed blood tests, blood transfusions were a major source of hepatitis transmission.

Hepatitis B is the lesser of the two viral evils, since it rarely goes on to cause chronic disease. We now have a vaccine against this virus that is standard for all children before they start school. In contrast, hepatitis C almost always becomes a silent, smoldering infection, typically showing up only after causing substantial liver damage. It has become a major trigger of liver cancer, here in the United States and around the world. It's estimated that there are some 4 million people chronically infected with hepatitis C in the United States alone, and the World Health Organization puts the number at more than 170 million worldwide. Until we develop a vaccine for this strain of hepatitis virus, too, these dismal numbers are unlikely to improve.

~*Other Pathogens*

One of the greatest surprises in medicine came with the discovery that it was a relatively unknown bacterium, *Helicobacter pylori*—and not stress or a type A personality—that causes most stomach ulcers. This same pathogen is also guilty of causing stomach cancer. Research in Japan, where this cancer is fairly common, shows that treating stomach ulcers with antibiotics prevents about half of stomach cancers and also plays an important role in the cancer's treatment.

The *H. pylori* bacterium, found in contaminated drinking water, takes hold of a vulnerable gastric lining and fosters chronic inflammation leading to injury and in some cases major ulceration. This persistent bacterial invasion is linked not only to the more common form of cancer of the stomach that originates in its lining cells but also to the less common and more easily treatable stomach lymphoma. As we've seen with other carcinogens, contributing factors can make the infection more virulent; these include older age, lower levels of gastric acidity, vitamin B deficiencies, and associated chemical carcinogens such as the nitrates and nitrites in cured meats.

Other pathogens are linked to cancer primarily because they cause a chronic and relentless state of inflammation, which is a risk factor for cancerous cell changes. In certain parts of the world, for example, liver parasites, such as the worm-like liver flukes, are tied to cancer of the bile duct; the water-borne parasite that causes schistosomiasis is associated with bladder cancer.

Finally, we come to animal viruses. Are they a threat to humans? Ordinarily animal viruses do not cross species barriers. But on occasion humans can become infected with animal viruses, and some have cancer-producing potential. This is a particular concern as we look to biological products for humans that have been made using animal serum or tissue. If stem cells, for example, are grown in animal cell cultures, or if animal organs or tissues are used for transplantation into humans, there is a risk of introducing novel pathogens into humans.

This is more than a theoretical concern, as time has taught us that viruses can adapt to life in more than one species. If the exposure is intimate enough, viruses prone to mutations anyway can learn to jump from animal to human. HIV came from primates. Less well known is the monkey virus SV40, which found its way into humans between 1955 and 1963 when certain batches of polio vaccine grown in monkey cells were found to be contaminated. Some researchers have linked chronic infection with the SV40 virus to the development of mesothelioma, non-Hodgkin's lymphoma, and bone and brain cancer because fragments of the virus have been identified in some of these tumors. Normal human tissue, however, can also carry the SV40 virus, presumably from the same source. The matter will not be resolved until members of the generation that got the contaminated polio virus move into their later years and we see whether the next generation shows a fall-off in these tumors.

I have no doubt that other pathogens will increasingly be recognized as cancer culprits in the years ahead. It is remarkable that in 2005 two classes of pathogens, HPV and hepatitis viruses B and C, for the first time made the long and infamous list of human carcinogens issued every year by the federal government's National Toxicology Program. More will follow.

This information at first glance might make us feel even more threatened and vulnerable: another whole class of carcinogens to fear. But this information is a good example of how we as individuals can strike a middle ground between ignoring risk and living in fear. The biological carcinogens show us that there is no one external risk to be fixated on, but rather several interacting ones—biological, chemical, and physical. And that offers a framework for protecting ourselves as we move through our lives faced with our own unique set of experiences. With regard to pathogens, once they are identified as a risk factor, control becomes possible—good hygiene, personal behavior, screening, and vaccination when available—that is mostly in our own hands. Armed with this information, I know I can have more meaningful discussions about cancer risks with my daughters and their friends than my parents' generation ever had. And that defines a grand new day for cancer prevention, both for us and for our children.

CHAPTER 7

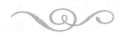

Making an Everyday Difference

EVEN THOUGH BUMMING A few cigarettes and soaking up some sunshine magnified with the help of a reflector were rituals of my college years, that didn't make it easier for me to watch my teenagers—despite all the school and parental attempts at brainwashing to the contrary—sneak away to a tanning parlor before the prom, or come home from a party smelling like smoke. Preaching cancer risk is still a tough sell among young people because illness, much less cancer, is just not on their minds. Furthermore, cancer prevention is easy to ignore, even for adults, because it's a matter of vigilance over long periods of time with no immediate or tangible threat. For our young people, cancer is mostly about their grandparents, occasionally about their parents. But hammering away relentlessly on these risks, even when their eyes seem to glaze over, while at the same time setting the right example, sooner or later finds its blessed rewards—the greatest being when their young frontal lobes mature to the point that they utter those priceless words: *Mom, you were right.*

Whatever our age, wherever we live, every single one of us has a stake in prevention. Certainly every cancer survivor does. But so does the patient who has just been given the diagnosis of cancer, and the healthy person who has any thoughts about living a long and healthy life. For any one of us, cancer prevention has no simple formula, but it starts with knowing the risks and then feeling deeply enough about the threats to embrace personal habits that avoid or lessen them. It's never too late to do so, but the sooner the better.

The first priorities are quite manageable: (1) Don't smoke, and avoid contact with secondhand smoke—even if it, sometimes seems rude. (2) Recognize sunburns as damage to skin. When outside, wear a hat and sunscreen. And stop worshiping tans. (3) Protect yourself against sexually transmitted diseases by thinking twice about having sex with any new partner and by practicing safe sex. If sexually active with multiple partners, both parties should be having regular screenings for STDs. These three behaviors will minimize the biggest and personally controllable environmental cancer risks and reduce cancer's toll on ourselves and our loved ones.

Next, pay attention to the less obvious and harder to quantify potential risks. For example, wash off fruit before you eat it, on the chance it may have traces of pesticide. Don't overdo it on the grilled meats, and try marinating or microwaving them briefly before grilling. Masks and gloves are in order when handling pesticides in the house or garden—or stop using these products altogether. Practice good hygiene, including faithful hand washing.

But decreasing your risk of cancer is about more than just avoiding hazard; it's also about embracing positive actions that can lower your cancer risk further still. And on this score, what you eat ranks overwhelmingly as number one.

Nutrition and Healthy Diet

The old English saying that we dig our grave with our spoon applies to our health in general and cancer in particular. Food does not cause cancer; rather, certain long-term dietary patterns can modestly increase or decrease the odds of getting cancer as we age. A diet rich in saturated fats is linked to an increased risk of cancer of the colon, prostate, uterine lining, and possibly breast and pancreas. High-salt diets and ones with lots of salt-preserved or nitrite-rich foods are linked to stomach cancer. Very hot drinks can increase the risk of cancer of the mouth, esophagus, and larynx. Moderate alcohol consumption may be good for the heart, but even modest imbibing has been linked to an increase in head and neck cancer and cancers of the liver and breast. Overdosing on red meat delivers a small risk for colon cancer.

Most of our understanding of the link between diet and cancer comes from studying the long-standing dietary habits of different societies. The Western countries, where diets are heavy with red meats, saturated fats, and refined sugars, suffer more breast, prostate, and colon cancer than those countries whose typical diets are low in saturated fats and higher in complex carbohydrates such as rice or pasta. When individuals of societies change dietary patterns over time, they provide an additional test for these linkages. For example, convincing associations between food and cancer have come from studies of populations in movement. When Japanese people migrate to California and adopt a more typically Western diet, their rates of breast and prostate cancer go up right along with heart disease, pointing a finger at the saturated fats in their new Western exposure.

But none of these studies speaks to the individual differences that we're coming to understand have so much to do with each person's health. The emerging power to identify genetic profiles among population groups will allow for a better grasp of the interaction between nutrition and individual metabolic patterns. Just as medicines are becoming more tailored to an individual's illness, so, too, will nutrition—more so as we recognize that food is not just calories or a means to soothe hunger, but a mix of chemicals essential to promoting health and warding off risks of chronic disease.

The terrible beauty of food is that how it tastes and satisfies can be a poor guide to how it functions in the body or how good it is for you personally. The main reason we ache for food is that it gives us energy. But every good thing has a price—as the body processes food as fuel, it spews out toxic by-products in the form of those DNA-oxidizing free radicals. But a healthy diet can also help provide a defense, in the form of antioxidant compounds, including some vitamins, that circulate in the blood and soak up the damaging free radicals.

Fruits and Vegetables

A nutritional bottom line is that a diet that lowers the metabolic risk of free radicals is good for health. And the best foods for that come from plants, not animals. Thus a simple principle of cancer prevention is to have a diet rich in fruits and vegetables—and that's a message for everyone, regardless of age or state of health.

Bruce Ames, who as noted earlier has made understanding the effect of chemicals on cancer development his life's career, believes that the public overestimates the potential risks of industrial chemicals, which appear only in trace amounts in the environment, while disregarding the single most important thing we can do for ourselves (along with avoiding tobacco), which is eating an abundance of fruits and vegetables. As he points out, the trivial amount of pesticides that gets onto produce (and which can usually be washed off) is the very thing that makes it affordable and accessible to everyone. And you don't have to buy organic to reap the anti-cancer benefits of fruits and vegetables.

What's clear is that Mother Nature offers us a means of protecting our genes through the natural chemicals of the garden. That does not mean I'm preaching a vegetarian diet. A delicious marbled beef, a slab of rich cheese, or a gooey chocolate sundae are all fine things—comfort foods, palate soothers, you name it. But they should be the treats. The bulk of the diet should come from plants, not animals. Time and time again scientific studies show that people who consume diets rich in varieties of fruits and vegetables cut their risk of getting most cancers. Fruits and vegetables are little factories pumping out all sorts of phytochemicals (*phyto*- means "plant"), not just the well-known micronutrients such as vitamins and minerals.

To give you a taste of this, let me list some of them. The flavonoids, which include thousands of chemicals called polyphenols, are present in all forms of flowers, fruits, vegetables, nuts, and tea. They are best known for their antioxidant properties as well as the ability of many of them to fight off viruses and fungal diseases. In this group we have the catechins, which are antioxidants and, in laboratory studies at least, also show the ability to induce deformed or cancerous cells to self-destruct. The carotenoids and retinoids—variations on vitamin A that provide rich red and yellow colors to vegetables—are also antioxidants. Add isothiocyanate to the list of plant preventives—this sulfur-containing compound helps the liver detoxify harmful molecules that get into the body. Other sulfur-containing plant compounds such as sulforaphane block the formation of carcinogenic nitrite, which otherwise would be produced by bacteria in the gut. Isoflavones, members of the flavonoid family and plentiful in soy products, have mild hormone-like effects in humans. By binding to the body's natural hormone receptors, they can mute the effects of the body's own natural estrogen and testosterone. (Lifelong high levels of estrogen are linked to breast cancer; testosterone, to prostate cancer.) We are only beginning to discover the nature of these numerous compounds and how they work in the body to explain the folklore that an apple a day—along with other fruits and vegetables—keeps the doctor away. They may someday be enhanced and deployed as specific therapies, but it takes nothing more than a nice salad to start enjoying their benefits today.

It's not that plants are philanthropists with a soft spot for the humans who eat them. They make these many chemicals as part of their own survival in the brutally competitive wild. But we can take advantage of their well-evolved chemical potions, as humans have for all of history. A good example of this is resveratrol, a polyphenol that hardy grape plants deploy to protect their delicate fruits from infection by bacteria and fungi, and from the heavy doses of sunlight that spur the plant's growth. Resveratrol can claim credit for much of wine's medicinal fame. Not surprisingly, given its role as a protectant, the grapes' defender is concentrated in the skin and shows up in large amounts in red wine. But it is made by all grapes of all colors, and also by blueberries, raspberries, cranberries, and peanuts. As discovered in the laboratory, resveratrol wields many powers, including inhibiting growth, reducing inflammation, and promoting apoptosis or suicide of human tumor cells growing in culture. As if this weren't enough, the multipurpose resveratrol has beneficial hormonal effects similar to soy products, and as a polyphenol, it is also a powerful antioxidant.

Not all fruits and vegetables are created equal when it comes to cancer protection. The top of the class includes blueberries, true champions of antioxidant strength, along with broccoli—no antioxidant slouch, but also a rich source of sulforaphane and the detoxifying isothiocyanates, present as well in cabbage and spinach. The yellow- and orange-colored fruits and vegetables—carrots, melons, pumpkin, sweet potatoes—are chock-full of carotenoids. Tomatoes, particularly in cooked form as tomato sauce and even ketchup, are veritable health stores, offering up 80 percent of the lycopenes (in the family of the colorful carotenoids), thought to reduce prostate, lung, and stomach cancer risk. Smokers with high blood carotenoid levels experience about half the expected rate of lung cancer—not a free pass on smoking, but certainly something all smokers should think about as they work to kick the addiction. Colorful citrus fruits and juices are also lush in carotenoids as well as high in the antioxidant vitamin C, believed to reduce the risk of almost every form of cancer. Cocoa and green tea are loaded with the powerful catechin EGCG (epigallocatechin-3-gallate). And even coffee has been recognized as a potential health food for its powerful supply of antioxidants.

Flavonoid-laden beans, particularly soy, have become health food celebrities because of their mildly estrogenic isoflavones, which compete with the stronger natural sex hormones. In many parts of Asia, where soy products are traditionally consumed in high amounts, the incidence of breast and prostate cancer is lower than in the West. There are also claims that soy protein inhibits both cancer invasion and spread. The isoflavones, scientists think, act like mild versions of SERMs—selective estrogen receptor modulators—such as tamoxifen and raloxifene, drugs that were designed expressly to prevent and treat breast cancer.

This litany of produce, laden with health- and repair-promoting phytochemicals, speaks to a critical dietary goal: variety. That's why the real deal comes with consuming the whole fruit or vegetable. A multivitamin pill or a jar of one or another concentrate can't replace the richness of a plant feast with all of its benefits, known and unknown. This reminds me of an experience I had at NIH. I was part of a launch of the National Cancer Institute's "five fruits and vegetables a day" campaign. In one appearance with then Secretary of Health and Human Services Louis Sullivan, we wrapped ourselves in aprons and stood before a colorful display of every imaginable variety of fruit and vegetable for the cameras, encouraging the viewers to get with the fruits-and-vegetables program. After we finished, one of the voices from the control room asked, with at least the pretense of sincerity, whether five glasses of wine would do. Sorry. Variety is of the essence.

Wine

Speaking of wine, red wine in particular has gotten a lot of attention for its health- and longevity-promoting properties because of a growing body of research on resveratrol, which is especially rich in the skin and seeds of grapes. Wine is also chock-full of other compounds with health benefits, such as catechin, epicatechin, and gallic acid. Numerous studies in the laboratory show beneficial effects of wine's polyphenols on tumor initiation, growth, and spread. Human studies are limited, but at least one performed on men showed that a glass of red wine a day cut in half their chance of getting prostate cancer, particularly in its more aggressive form. Although the anti-cancer effects are related to the non-alcoholic chemicals, during the fermentation process it is the alcohol that extracts the polyphenols from the grapes' seeds and skins and concentrates them in the final libation.

There is a gentle caution here: wine may be a rich fruit concentrate, filled with beneficial chemicals, but that does not make it a health elixir. Population studies show that the risk of cancers of the liver, head and neck, and breast start going up with increasing daily alcohol consumption—and that includes wine—starting at the equivalent of just one glass of wine per day. As in all things, moderation.

Whole Grains and Fiber

Fiber is a friend of the heart and the gut and is another reason that fruits and vegetables are healthy choices. Grains, fruits, and vegetables have lots of the soluble form of fiber, which reduces cholesterol and slows down glucose absorption into the bloodstream, bringing particular benefit to the heart. It is the insoluble form of fiber present in brans, whole grains, and the pulp and skin of fruits and vegetables that is believed to bring cancer protection. By soaking up toxic products made by the bacterial breakdown of food in the intestine, and by generally keeping things moving through the system, fiber keeps toxic waste products from lingering in the gut. Proven benefits include fewer colon polyps and thus less risk of colon cancer.

I hope you are at least a bit persuaded about plant magic. Prevention is more than an intellectual experience, however. It is about taste and choice. You choose what you put in your mouth and often it is just a matter of habit and convenience. The only way to get serious about this is to first start counting. Though the number has been slowly increasing, only about 40 percent of Americans consume the currently recommended levels of at least two fruits and three vegetables per day. I have gotten into this habit and it just means you have to plan ahead. Make the right choices at the grocery store, when you open the refrigerator or a can of soup, stuff your lunch bag, or place your order at a fast-food counter or a fancy restaurant. It's the little choices, made day in and day out, that add up. When given the choice, choose a glass of fruit or vegetable juice rather than a soda pop. Think apple or a handful of baby carrots rather than a chocolate chip cookie or donut. Think long years of health and vitality rather than the alternative.

Dietary Fats and Oils

That brings us to fats—a topic of some controversy when it comes to cancer risk. There is nothing wrong with fats per se; it's just that in our national daily diet we consume too many of them, particularly saturated fats and the artificially saturated fats now famously known as trans fats. The process of hydrogenation, which produces virtually all of the trans fats we consume, is a modern-day invention, designed to convert perfectly healthy plant oils into solid fat. That way, it's less apt to get rancid, and it can take the place of animal fat in shelf-stable products such as the nearly immortal cookies and crackers that can lie in wait in your larder for years without spoiling. Ironically, trans fats in the form of stick margarine were once heavily marketed as the healthy substitute for butter. I well recall the many lunches and dinners at the American Heart Association in which margarine was pressed into yellow rosettes as part of the heart-healthy diet. We now know better. As a general rule, if the fat is solid, go easy on it. (There is the exception of the new heart-healthy butter-like products now on the market that are solid but contain no trans fats.)

Evidence continues to accumulate that low-fat diets are not just good for the heart but also associated with lower risk for colon and prostate cancer—and maybe cancer of the breast. But the merits of these associations have been hotly debated and are hard to prove. I got a taste of the fat controversy shortly after we launched the Women's Health Initiative in 1992, which I began during my tenure as director of NIH. This was the largest scientifically controlled clinical trial of women's wellness and health risks ever conducted, involving more than 150,000 women to be studied for more than fifteen years. One dimension of the trial looked at the effects of fat in the diet on both heart disease and cancer. That fat in the diet increases the risk of breast cancer had been suspected, but skeptics at the time felt the study could not be done, particularly in a diverse population with different eating habits—an attitude that has historically retarded nutrition studies in general. (It is also why food fads take on such credence.) Even more, the critics rejected the idea that a breast cancer–fat connection was plausible, though they were confident that a low-fat diet would reduce the risks of colon cancer and heart disease. Reducing fat in the diet from 37 to 20 percent of calories consumed, which has been promoted as ideal for all Americans, was a very tall order.

The Women's Health Initiative controlled trial compared usual diet with one designed to reduce total fat consumption by almost half in a cross section of American women over the age of fifty. One discovery was that despite the best efforts of a motivated group of women, reducing fat in a regular Western diet to 20 percent of total calories was not achievable or sustainable for most people. But what the study also showed clearly was that you *can* significantly reduce fat in the diet and sustain it over an extended period of time. Women in the intervention group, who were eating from fat-reduction menus and receiving regular nutritional counseling and group support, reduced their baseline level of fat intake from 37 to 24 percent, which then leveled off at about 29 percent for much of the eight years of the study. That's an accomplishment, since the women stuck to a level of dietary fat significantly lower than where they had been or than the control group of similar women. This was the case despite the fact that the control group, in what doctors call a secular effect, actually dropped its fat intake on its own—likely in response to general population awareness of healthier eating. The intervention group, in response to regular prompts and encouragement, also consumed one more fruit or vegetable a day, just reaching the minimum of five recommended.

And the effects on cancer? At first glance, the findings were a disappointment. After seven years, the incidence of colon cancer and heart disease was the same in both groups. If one looks at the data more closely, however, there is a consistent trend toward a modest reduction in breast cancer: breast cancer incidence was lowered by 9 percent in the group of women that consumed less fat. (It came close—a 10 percent reduction would have been statistically significant.) And the decrease in risk was significant among women who entered the study with the highest levels of fat in their diets. Similarly, the modest trend toward lower levels of invasive colon cancer takes on more importance when it is coupled with an additional finding: women consuming diets with less fat and one extra fruit or vegetable had significantly fewer pre-malignant polyps— harbingers of colon cancer that can take a decade or more to turn cancerous.

Thus the overall reduction in these cancers, and the pattern of reduction, cannot be dismissed. The study interval of eight years was also relatively short when one considers the long lead time for most cancers. If anything, it's reasonable to conclude that dietary modification that is longer and starts before age fifty or sixty is going to offer greater benefit.

The Women's Health Initiative study is an important step in searching for a connection between total dietary fat and cancer in a large and diverse population. We still need follow-up studies to determine how different types of fats influence health and cancer risk. Fats can be of plant, fish, or animal origin; they become incorporated into the structure of cells, such as the cell membrane, and play key roles in metabolism that influence core functions of the immune system and blood vessel regulation. There is a growing body of information to show that fats don't all weigh in equally, even among the unsaturated group: the monounsaturated fats of olive oil and the omega-3s of fish oil seem to bring positive health benefits not seen with other forms of unsaturated fat.

As for fats and breast cancer specifically, evidence continues to stoke the belief that there is a connection between the two. In May 2005, the Women's Intervention Nutrition Study, conducted by the American Health Foundation and involving thirty-seven medical centers around the country, showed that a low-fat diet reduced recurrence rates of breast cancer by 24 percent over five years in more than 2,400 women with similar lifestyles. The unexpected result was that women with breast cancer that was negative for estrogen receptors saw an even higher reduction—42 percent. That variants of a particular tumor react differently to a cancer risk reduction effort gives further weight to the notion of personalized prescriptions—for food as well as medicine.

Importantly, the Women's Health Initiative shows that prospective diet studies are doable in a reasonable length of time—and we'd better get on with them. Until now they have simply not been part of the nutritional landscape, leaving a void for anyone who shops, cooks, or eats. As we wait for more complete data, the common-sense formula still holds: go easy on saturated fats and increase your intake of fruits and vegetables, and based on your own personal diet, consider dietary supplements.

Dietary Supplements

Some nutrients with outstanding potential to reduce cancer risk simply cannot be provided at sufficient levels by even the best diet of fruits and vegetables. The general rule for supplements, however, is that they are just that: supplements, and not replacements.

Vitamins and Minerals

Historically, the medical community has been down on food supplements and has resisted even the daily multivitamin. "Expensive urine" is a common scorn laid on daily vitamin pill intake. But time has mellowed that view, and many doctors now recommend a multivitamin a day, plus supplemental calcium. Vitamins' role in cancer prevention is still under investigation in laboratory and clinical studies, but the evidence so far is that many vitamins play a part in nature's defense against genes going wrong.

Members of the vitamin A family of retinoids can be anti-cancer agents for a variety of tumors, including prostate cancer, breast cancer, acute promyelogenous leukemia, thyroid cancer, head and neck cancer, and certain brain and lung cancers. Vitamin A affects the expression of a variety of genes and pushes cells from a more primitive state to a more differentiated one. This property has led to using high doses of vitamin A analogues such as isotretinoin (Accutane) as an adjunct in chemotherapy. But results from clinical studies on the prevention of cancer with vitamin A have been mixed.

Part of the difficulty in sorting out the risks and benefits of vitamin A compounds is that these chemicals have many possible function in the body, with a narrow range between how much is beneficial and how much is toxic, particularly to the liver. In fetal development, either too much or too little vitamin A can cause major congenital malformations. Because of this, the FDA has fairly restrictive policies on access to isotretinoin, and it is unlikely that the drug at any dose will be useful as a cancer preventive.

Next in the alphabet are the B vitamins, and in particular folic acid, which plays a protective role in fetal development. Taking folate supplements before becoming pregnant virtually eliminates spina bifida, a debilitating birth defect of the lower spinal cord. Prenatal folic acid supplements have also been shown to decrease childhood cancer risk by as much as 60 percent. In adults, folate has been proven to lessen colon cancer risk. Folate is plentiful in spinach, citrus fruits, and tomatoes, as well as in fortified flour, breads, and cereals, but to ensure getting enough folic acid into your system you still need a supplement of around 400 micrograms a day, which is the amount found in most multivitamins.

Vitamins C and E have been pushed for their antioxidant, anticancer effects, but studies of the individual supplements taken in isolated pill form have failed to show convincing benefit against cancer. We do know that vitamin C boosts the immune system, which is a good thing, and in several studies seems to ward off pre-cancerous changes in the cervix. Two major studies, however, showed that beta-carotene and vitamin A supplements (as opposed to carotenoids from fruits and vegetables) actually increased the likelihood of lung cancer among smokers, almost as if they were feeding the tumor's growth. This is a lingering concern for all cancers—remember that tumors feed off their victim's own blood supply and have their own requirements for good nutrition—which argues against any kind of megavitamin use in patients who are undergoing cancer treatment. Vitamin E, another antioxidant, which also has an aspirin-like effect on platelets (making the blood thinner), has been touted for its anticancer effect. But again, as a stand-alone it has failed in repeated studies to show protective benefits for either heart disease or cancer. Taking supplements of vitamins A and E beyond the recommended doses in a daily multivitamin is generally not advised.

The sleeper vitamin and mineral just may be vitamin D and calcium. We think bones when we hear of calcium and vitamin D, but there may be more to this mineral and its vitamin companion when it comes to cancer. In the laboratory vitamin D promotes normal cell development and makes many cancer cell lines undergo apoptosis. Other studies show it has anti-angiogenic properties. What is provocative is that in large population studies, vitamin D and calcium are linked to a lower risk of colon, prostate, breast, and ovarian cancer. And reports going back to the 1930s have shown that those who live in places with more sunlight, which promotes vitamin D production by the skin, have less cancer.

The controlled trial of supplemental vitamin D and calcium carried out in the Women's Health Initiative, however, failed to demonstrate its anti-cancer properties. Bone health was clearly improved over a seven-year period and hip fractures were reduced, but the study detected no evidence of an anti-cancer effect. More recent research suggests that in order to see an anti-cancer effect, even higher levels of vitamin D than were used in the Women's Health Initiative are required—perhaps as high as 1,000 IU or more. Right now vitamin D biology is hot, and there is growing interest in its effects beyond bone health, particularly on both cancer and the nervous system.

Meanwhile, nutritional advice is straightforward: calcium and vitamin D are needed for our bones anyway, and American diets generally run short on them, because our dietary calcium and vitamin D come mostly from milk products, a dairy habit often left behind in childhood. Since most people are not going to or simply can't drink a quart of milk a day, and are not always able to take in the ten minutes a day of sunshine to generate vitamin D in the skin, the average adult diet calls for supplements. That means a combination of 800 IU of vitamin D plus 500 to 1,000 milligrams of calcium, depending on just how shy your daily diet is of the recommended levels of calcium. For example, post-menopausal women need 1,200 to 1,500 milligrams of calcium per day; the average intake among American women is about half that. Yes, we are a calcium-malnourished country.

Trace Minerals

Unlike calcium, which the body uses in bulk, many of the minerals that contribute to the body's well-being come from food and water in trace amounts. Selenium, a mineral that is needed in only the smallest amounts by the body, has drawn attention as a tumor fighter, particularly against prostate cancer, as well as colon, esophageal, and lung cancers. A major study from Cornell University showed that both the occurrence of and mortality from these tumors fell when participants took selenium supplements. But nutrition is complex, and the results of other studies have not been so clear. Research is further hampered by the limited knowledge of just how much of this trace element any one individual gets in his or her diet. Agricultural scientists have seen promising results inhibiting tumors in animals using selenium-enriched vegetables such as onions and broccoli. But here again the problem is that too much selenium is toxic, causing fatigue, hair loss, and even a weakening of the immune system. Nonetheless, selenium has a following among some in the health food community, and until further studies are completed the jury will remain out. If you're inclined to take it, heed the nutritional guidance of the National Academy of Sciences and do not consume more than 400 micrograms per day—which includes the 100 micrograms or so that come in a customary diet.

Other Nutritional Supplements

As we delve deeper into plants' wisdom, we see a wealth of cancer-fighting micronutrients still locked up in the roots and leaves of fruits and vegetables, as well as in flowers and herbs—substances that can be labeled broadly as nutriceuticals. Until they are sufficiently characterized and studied for their mechanism of therapeutic benefits, doses, and toxicity, they will stay largely untapped. What is the chemical magic behind the blueberry? Can it be tapped by an extract or do you need the whole fruit? Is there a benefit to taking a resveratrol supplement rather than consuming a pound of grapes? And how about that health food favorite, green tea? Let me use green tea as one example of the evolution from natural product to chemopreventive dietary supplement.

Green tea has been a medicinal potion for thousands of years. Laden with flavonoids, the leaves are touted as offering protection against both coronary disease and cancer. But just how green tea works its wonders in the prevention or treatment of individual disease has been a mystery. Dr. Thomas Gasiewicz of the University of Rochester Medical Center has identified some unique anti-cancer properties in one of the antioxidant components of green tea, the catechin molecule called epigallocatechin-3-gallate, or EGCG. EGCG targets a specific heat shock protein (discussed in Chapter 4) in the cancer cell, a normal stress protein known as HSP 90, which is critical to survival of all cells, cancerous or otherwise. EGCG does battle with that hijacked stress protein in cancer cells by binding to it and knocking it out of commission.

But you have to drink quite a lot of tea to get enough EGCG to do any good—probably somewhere between three and ten cups a day. Because of its bitterness and the caffeine load of that much tea, this can be hard to do. So it's not surprising that a detailed analysis of numerous studies of green tea as a preventive against cancer in tens of thousands of patients led the Food and Drug Administration to conclude that there is no credible evidence to allow makers of green tea to assert that health claim. Before we bury green tea, however, some scientists believe we have to look at the potential benefit of a concentrated green tea extract, a richer source of EGCG, to deliver a meaningful dose of this compound and free it from the side effects of overdosing on the brew.

It's a big task to move from natural substance to the medicine cabinet. There are few financial incentives to underwrite the same kind of clinical studies that we expect for pharmaceuticals. The studies that do exist are hampered by not being sure of the right dose for benefit (or the toxic dose), even if there is a good idea of what result can be achieved in a cell culture or animal laboratory.

The world of chemoprevention using plant-based and over-the-counter nutriceuticals is a young science with enormous promise. But inexpensive food extracts have limited sources of research support, and much of the work is conducted in schools of agriculture that do not have ready access to clinical research. Without the patent protection that would attract large pharmaceutical houses, the field categorically needs greater public support. Nutritional research is happening in a spotty way in disease-focused institutes at NIH, and within the center at NIH devoted to complementary medicines. But the pace is slow.

That slow pace will keep functional foods in knowledge limbo, even those already singled out for their health benefits beyond basic nutrition. Yet the pharmacy shelves and health food stores will continue to be stocked with nutriceuticals, be they antioxidants, megavitamins, minerals, fish oil supplements, or targeted hormone modifiers. The public will consume them but not know for sure if they should.

This reality only fuels my long-standing belief that the nutritional sciences need more research investment, something that public health demands. I'm now convinced that would be best and enduringly served by forming a National Institute of Nutrition Research within the NIH. Not only would a nutrition institute have its own designated research dollars and bring the nutritional sciences and their basic and clinical researchers into the fold of traditional medicine, but it would also provide a platform for development of future researchers, for education of the public, and for public advocacy of a field all too neglected.

Exercise and Body Weight

Humans are just not meant to be slugs. Yet so much of our creative energy has gone into ways of cutting back on physical work that the modern environment we have built for ourselves discourages bodily motion. Cars take us most places, not our legs; between computers and TV screens we barely have to move about our workspace or our home to be entertained or get things done. Yet however it is tallied, exercising our limbs and working our hearts are of prime benefit to mental and physical health. The cancer prevention arena is no exception. The link between reduced cancer risk and exercise has long been recognized for cancer of the colon, and there the connection is clear. Gut motility is improved by moving around, and toxic waste is pushed along faster, giving gut mucosa less exposure to its carcinogens. But more recent studies have also shown that women who exercise face lower rates of recurrence of a prior breast cancer. And those who have less sedentary lives experience fewer cancers overall. Exercise is a mood booster, too, resulting in less depression and a greater sense of control and optimism—an important part of keeping the immune system active and robust.

How much exercise is enough? You do not need to be a marathon runner. The best formula is to engage in some form of exercise that you enjoy for about thirty minutes a day at least five days a week. Sure, an hour would be better, and so would working out every day, but don't let the ideal get in the way of the pretty good. And it doesn't have to be done all at once. What's key is to think about it, and keep track of your activities, so that exercise becomes part of your daily routine.

Of Calories and Cancer

One intriguing health discovery is the protective value of very low-calorie diets. We first learned this from studying rats whose calories were cut by more than half, resulting in consistently longer life spans. These findings conformed to observations in humans linking longevity to caloric intake. How can this be? The most popular theory is that fewer calories mean less oxidation is going on and therefore fewer destructive free radicals are floating around and doing damage to DNA. There could also be a more direct connection to blood sugar.

Consuming fewer calories overall results in fewer and less severe sugar spikes—the sudden jolts of sugar that call insulin into play. Cutting back on the glucose spikes should also cut back on blood levels of insulin-like growth factors. These are chemicals your body makes that stimulate cell proliferation and block apoptosis. High levels of these growth factors have been associated with breast, prostate, and colon cancer. Another factor may be excess steroid hormones manufactured by fat cells, where the extra calories are stored. Whatever the reason, there is something to the observation that it's better to consume fewer calories in your day rather than more. That goes beyond the fact that fewer calories means less body fat, and obesity is a risk factor for certain cancers.

Obesity has gotten a lot of national attention of late, in part because America is steadily getting fatter. But the link between excess weight and cancer risk is not as clear as it has been, for example, for high blood pressure and stroke. However, for certain kinds of cancer, the evidence is mounting. Tumors of the colon, prostate, breast, uterus, kidney, and esophagus seem to disproportionately hit those lugging around too many extra pounds. In 1982, the American Cancer Society began the Cancer Prevention Study II, which examined the relationship between cancer mortality and weight in 900,000 Americans followed for at least sixteen years. Cancer mortality increased as BMI (body mass index) increased over 30. For those individuals with BMIs over 40, mortality was 50 percent greater. You can determine your own BMI by using calculators readily available online. Or you can calculate it yourself by knowing your height and weight: multiply your weight in pounds times 703, and divide that number by your height in inches squared. For most body types normal is less than 25. It's a number worth knowing, as the American Cancer Society blames elevated BMI for about 20 percent of female and 14 percent of male cancer deaths.

As for watching that weight, let me add a word of cancer caution here about how *not* to do it. Avoid fad diets. They are seductive in that they preach an easy way to wage the battle of the bulge, but you will never win the war this way, since the fat comes back when the diet ends. Some of these diets also proclaim heart benefits. For some reason, a lowering-your-cancer-risk diet just doesn't sell. But what's worse is that many of the fad diets might be viewed as pro-cancer, not the opposite. Look at the Atkins diet. Not only does it sell itself on its high-saturated-fats-are-good theme, but its low-carb stance pushes beneficial fruits, vegetables, grains, and fiber right off the table—exactly what you should *not* do if you are trying to reduce your cancer risk.

What makes the full range of cancer prevention habits compelling is that all together they bring a broader health value. A low-fat diet high in fruits and vegetables, supplemental calcium and vitamin D if your diet is low on them, healthy body weight, restricted sun exposure, and saying no to tobacco bring benefits to heart and bone health as well as lowering one's risk for cancer. That's good value, and good reason to get on with it.

CHAPTER 8

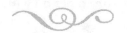

Working with Your Doctor

I N A WORLD IN which having the same primary care doctor forever has gone the way of the buggy whip, it's important to remember that you have a better sense of your lifetime risk of getting cancer than does any one of your doctors. The new and emerging culture of consumer-directed health care will work only if patients themselves maintain up-to-date copies of their health history and those of their family members. Tallying your personal risk for common illnesses will be part of the task.

Radiation exposure is a good example of what I mean. We all should keep track of how many X-rays we (and our children) have had over the years. As I mentioned in Chapter 6, the risk is a cumulative one. Ask your dentist whether you really need those dental X-rays every single year; I'm not so sure you do. And keep track of those CT scans. The FDA estimates that a single abdominal CT scan carries the radiation impact of 500 chest X-rays. Physicist David Brenner and his colleagues point out that a twenty-minute CT scan can deliver the same radiation exposure as if you were standing just a mile and a half from the atom bomb explosion at Hiroshima. Both of these are chilling thoughts, and ones that should certainly cool any interest in those total body scans now being offered commercially to screen healthy people for hidden illness. Whenever X-rays or imaging studies are being considered, it's legitimate to discuss with your doctor your prior radiation exposure. You should also talk about diet, exercise, unusual environmental exposures at home or work, and options for cancer screening. Preventive oncology is a new science, and the proper formula needs to be tailored to the individual patient. As we learn more about the value of chemoprevention, these discussions will become a routine part of primary care.

Chemoprevention

Preventing serious disease by taking prescription drugs, be they ones to make your blood pressure normal, lower your cholesterol, or keep your blood thin, is an established practice unique to modern-day medicine. Such practices have been slow to penetrate the field of oncology in large part because we have known so little about the biology of cancer development. At the National Cancer Institute, pioneers of this approach work in a relatively small Division of Cancer Prevention led by cancer researcher Peter Greenwald, who has pursued this work for over twenty years. Covering the full gamut of diet, alternative therapies, and early cancer screening, its most controversial efforts over the years involved research using drugs as preventive agents to lower cancer risk.

This concept of a preventive medicine is not so alien if one considers that preventive surgery is a time-tested approach to dodging the cancer bullet in patients known to have, or be at, high risk for rare forms of familial cancer of the colon, in which oncologists advise a total colectomy before age forty. Although the magnitude of the threat is not as great, some women opt for prophylactic removal of their breasts or ovaries if they have a strong family history of the disease appearing at a young age in their mother or sisters, or if that link is further confirmed through genetic testing. Compared to preventive surgery, chemoprevention seems like a reasonable alternative.

The field of preventive oncology has been stymied, however, because of limitations in our predictive abilities. While we can assess risk in broadly defined populations, it's harder to come up with risk measures for any one woman. For example, women who have a family history of the disease or who have their children late in life have a small increase in breast cancer. To assess the value of chemoprevention you need to offer it only to those individuals in whom there is a substantial risk that would justify any side effects that are bound to come with chronic medication. What brought some confidence that this could be done, and with success, was a major study, led by the Division of Cancer Prevention at the National Cancer Institute, using the drug tamoxifen to lower high-risk women's chances of getting breast cancer. The tamoxifen study was, nonetheless, a bear to accomplish.

Tamoxifen was originally designed as a cancer treatment that blocked the specific kind of estrogen receptor that is native to breast tissue. Some but not all breast cancers are replete with estrogen receptors, and their stimulation spurs cancer progression. Decades ago it was routine to remove the ovaries as part of the treatment of breast cancer because of this association, making for a pretty rough time for women back then: radical mastectomy followed by pelvic surgery to remove their ovaries. In women of childbearing age, that ordeal also brought on early menopause, with its own risks and discomforts.

Tamoxifen changed this. The drug blocks the breast estrogen receptors selectively, acting like an anti-estrogen on breast tissue but stimulating receptors in other organs such as bone, where it brings estrogenic benefits. This so-called designer hormone, also known as a selective estrogen receptor modulator, or SERM, quickly became routine as an adjunct to chemotherapy for breast cancer, where its use led to a surprising observation. Women who have cancer in one breast are known to have a greater chance of getting cancer in their other breast. Tamoxifen cut that risk by at least 30 percent. That discovery led to the idea that women at high risk for breast cancer might be spared the disease if they used a SERM.

The tamoxifen study, known officially as the Breast Cancer Prevention Trial, seemed like a natural when I heard about it as NIH director back in 1991, no doubt because of my own faith in prevention using medication, which is so well practiced in cardiology. Since estrogen is a known risk for breast cancer, lowering its impact selectively on the breast in high-risk women made enormous sense. The team that led the effort was an impressive one, including NCI's Leslie Ford and Peter Greenwald, along with Salim Yusuf, a preventive cardiologist then working with the National Heart, Lung, and Blood Institute. The researchers radiated excitement that the tamoxifen study could radically change our thinking about breast cancer and the prevention of cancer in general. Plus, as Salim enthusiastically pointed out, this estrogen-like drug, tamoxifen, was likely to benefit bone and, by lowering cholesterol, perhaps even the heart. There was a concern, however, identified from the start: the drug also stimulates estrogen receptors in the uterus and therefore increases the risk of cancer of the uterus, a typically slow-growing and easily cured malignancy. But about 2 women in 10,000 per year taking the drug developed a more aggressive and life-threatening form of uterine cancer. The estrogen-like effect of tamoxifen also increases the risk of blood clots. Patients would be monitored for both of these possible complications.

The study enrolled more than 13,000 healthy but high-risk women to embark on a five-year course of tamoxifen—and the study was controversial almost from the start. Did a theoretical benefit justify known risks? Dr. Ford tenaciously shepherded this study through its ups and downs as it came under mounting pressure from some activists and members of Congress, many of whom wanted to stop the study cold. In October 1992, a full six months into the study, she and I sat together at a packed congressional hearing conducted by a House Government Operations subcommittee that tore into the trial and into both of us. Dr. Ford was the one who led the federal study; I was the one who had the authority to stop it.

The central argument against the trial was that a drug with serious side effects, however rare, should not be given to healthy people for what was "a highly questionable benefit." I was puzzled by the arguments, as some doctors were already prescribing tamoxifen for prevention without the benefit of a rigorous trial. As for the concern about giving drugs to healthy people, we do that already with vaccinations and with the many drugs we cardiologists prescribe like water—all of which have a risk of complications. Though rancorous, the hearing ended with our assurances that the study did monitor all women closely and that its consent forms would be beefed up even more to emphasize the drug's risks. Despite the controversy and some bad press, NIH continued on with the trial—and women across the country continued to enroll in what was, at the time, the largest cancer prevention study ever. Their enrollment paid off.

The results came in early. Women on tamoxifen had roughly 50 percent fewer diagnoses of both invasive and in-situ breast cancers when compared to women taking placebo pills. An added, but not surprising, benefit from taking this estrogen-like drug was its positive effect on bone health: there were far fewer fractures of the hip, wrist, and spine. The study was released with considerable fanfare in 1998. Cancer researchers hailed this effort as nothing short of a landmark achievement, establishing that cancer could be prevented with drugs.

The enthusiasm continued as large studies from abroad came in with similar or even better results, leading the FDA to approve tamoxifen for prevention of breast cancer in high-risk women. Updated results from women who finished the study seven years later, in 2005, showed that tamoxifen cuts the risk of both invasive and noninvasive breast cancer even after patients stop taking the drug. Thus the benefit does not require lifelong use, and doctors now advise women not to take tamoxifen for more than five years.

The findings of the tamoxifen trial spurred interest in other designer estrogens. Evista (raloxifene) is one that selectively blocks estrogen receptors in the breast but also in the uterus, eliminating the uterine cancer risk. In 1999 the FDA approved Evista for use in women with osteoporosis because of its estrogen-like effects on bone. In 2006, after completion of a major clinical trial of its use in women at high risk for breast cancer, the drug also gained official approval as a breast cancer chemopreventive.

But chemoprevention puts front and center a key issue for any prophylactic medication used over a long period of time: that risks must be weighed as well as benefits. When the tamoxifen results were released, Dr. Ford stressed that this preventive strategy brought rare but predicted side effects, including blood clots and cancer of the uterus. Though the complications could not be predicted for any one woman, the risks occurred mainly in women fifty years of age and older. So for some high-risk women under fifty, the benefits can outweigh the risks.

The decision to embark on any form of drug prevention therapy for cancer ultimately involves this kind of individual calculation of benefit and risk. Look at the studies of the anti-inflammatory drugs Vioxx and Celebrex. Members of the COX-2 inhibitor family of anti-inflammatory agents, they decrease the risk of pre-malignant polyp formation in the colon. The long-term chemoprevention studies demonstrated, however, an unexpected increase in heart attacks, primarily in older patients. But the dramatic reduction in the precancerous growths, close to 70 percent in one study, persuades many doctors to prescribe the therapy to patients who have no heart risk factors but have shown aggressive pre-cancerous polyp formation—provided they know the potential side effects.

Therein lies a crucial lesson: whether it's a new or old drug or one of the many emerging natural products from food mentioned earlier, the very effect that brings a benefit can also bring a measure of harm. The hope is that modern gene-targeted medicine will change that. The emerging fields of pharmacogenomics for drugs and nutrigenomics for nutrients offer the means to tailor drugs or diet to your genes. Combining genomics, proteomics, and the even newer metabolomics—which analyzes the soup of molecules that results from your metabolic activity—might even offer the formula for a personalized and integrated daily drug and dietary bill of fare. This is, of course, some way off, but companies are already forming to try to get a jump on crafting DNA diets. And most large pharmaceutical houses see genomics as a way to detect ahead of time those at risk for a negative drug side effect. But along with this promise, we should not forget the best cancer chemopreventives we have so far: the mighty mix of natural chemicals found in fruits and vegetables.

Cancer Screening

Since mutations and malignant cell transformations are not going to disappear from the human experience, and since these cells do not show their hand until they are already well entrenched, waiting for cancer symptoms to develop is waiting too long. For now, the only way to prevent cancer's harm and minimize the need for debilitating therapy is to find the malignancy early, when it is small and localized. In fact, the strength or weakness of the diagnostic screening tools that we have in our medical arsenal today closely tracks our success in curing and controlling any given cancer.

But success also tracks a person's willingness to embark on a disciplined program of cancer screening, a rite of passage into middle age that, once initiated, should go on for the rest of your life. Signing up for the program is something only you can do. Spend the time, accept the inconvenience, and put up with a little discomfort or anxiety. Sure, it's hard to go to a doctor when you feel well, to think about a possible illness when you are healthy. It's easy to forget to do a monthly breast exam or scan your skin for funny-looking moles. It might seem like a drag to spend time, money, or mental focus all because of a small, theoretical risk and undergo medical tests for cancer screening that might turn up the wrong answer. But there is no choice if we want to be part of winning the war on cancer.

For Women: Mammogram Wars and Better Pap Smears

Breast self-exam, a yearly doctor's exam, and a mammogram are the three pillars of breast cancer screening. The limitation of manual breast exams is that they can only find what can be felt. They miss the small tumors and the in-situ microscopic clusters of cancer cells not large enough to form lumps, signaled only by specks of calcium on the mammogram. The current guideline is that women should have a mammogram every one to two years beginning at age forty, or at age thirty-five if there's a strong family history. However, getting to this recommendation hasn't been easy.

For almost two decades, many public health advocates and the U.S. Preventive Services Task Force in the Department of Health and Human Services advised against mammograms for women in their forties; the thinking was that although mammograms detected tumors earlier, there was no solid proof (through randomized clinical trials) that they saved lives. At the same time the American Cancer Society and the National Cancer Institute promoted them for younger women, which sent a mixed public message. (There was agreement that evidence was strong enough to advocate the use of routine mammograms in women over age fifty.) In 1997, a National Institutes of Health consensus conference weighed in against screening women in their forties, and at least briefly the National Cancer Institute went along—leading to an outcry from doctors and women alike, and turning the differences of opinion into a public mammogram war.

The argument for limiting mammograms in women under fifty may seem arcane, but is worth understanding since it's the same argument that is applied again and again to newer tests that screen healthy populations for unsuspected disease. Here it is: for mammography to detect five early cancers and save one life in women in their forties, radiologists must screen 2,500 women. That costs money. And since mammograms have a false positive rate of 10 percent, 250 healthy women will face pain, anxiety, and sometimes a biopsy to identify those five women with cancer. That costs even more money. Some policy makers, particularly those with an eye on what's best for the overall public health, see this as too low a yield, and a waste of medical resources that would be better spent elsewhere.

Unless yours is the life that's been saved, that is—and that is what saved early mammograms. Women and their doctors forced the issue into the public and political arena, and the NCI reversed its course, finally going along with the American Cancer Society's unwavering position that forty-something women should be screened regularly for breast cancer with mammograms. Doctors who had been ordering mammograms for women according to the older guidelines, and women who demanded them, were vindicated. Unfortunately, many women are still confused by the recommendation whiplash.

There are other methods of screening for early breast cancer. Ultrasound and MRIs are sometimes used if there is a suspicious or equivocal area on a regular mammogram. Another technique for finding early breast tumors, refined and advanced by breast cancer surgeon Dr. Susan Love—though not routinely used at present—is ductal lavage. It's designed as a kind of Pap smear for the superficial cells that line the milk ducts of the breast where most cancers originate. Using a special catheter, saline is injected into the milk ducts through the nipples and then sucked back into the catheter, and the fluid is screened for cancerous cells. This test does not replace the mammogram, and if it finds abnormal cells, it does not provide information as to their extent or whether cancer cells are invasive. Lavage might eventually be a means for administering drugs directly into the ducts to ward off cancer and destroy any pre-cancerous cells that may be lurking.

Pap smears are a great success story that proves screening for the earliest of disease can save lives and preserve quality of life. Though invasive cancer of the cervix has plummeted in most developed countries because routine Pap smears starting at about eighteen years of age are a standard part of women's health care, cervical cancer remains common in women who have no access to such screening. According to the World Health Organization, this invasive disease afflicts about 450,000 women each year and takes the lives of more than half of them, making it the number two cancer killer of women overall. Compare that to the United States, where in the 1930s the incidence of deaths from cervical cancer exceeded deaths from lung and breast cancer combined. Thinking about this another way, 80 percent of the women who died of this cancer back then would be saved from such a brutal demise today.

With Pap smears, doctors search for disfigured or frankly cancerous cells in scrapings from the cervix. But with modern technology they can also detect the presence of HPV in those cells and distinguish benign viral strains from cancer-producing ones. The presence of the oncogenic strains of HPV identifies women who need closer long-term monitoring.

For Men: Prostate-Specific Antigen (PSA)

The test for prostate-specific antigen, or PSA, came into clinical practice as a way to follow the course of cancer in those who already had the disease. A protein that is secreted by cells in the prostate, PSA is elevated even in early prostate cancer. Through clinical experience doctors learned that a PSA test could signal cancer long before signs or symptoms of the disease showed up, and even before a physician could detect it by performing a digital rectal exam.

Clinical experience over many years has turned this test into a "must" preventive screen, and most doctors will tell you that lives have been saved by finding the disease in its easiest-to-treat—and easiest-to-cure—stage. The American Cancer Society now recommends that doctors offer men this test along with a digital rectal exam yearly, starting at age fifty. If a man has a strong family history of the disease or if he is African American, a group with a particularly high risk for prostate cancer, he should first be screened at age forty-five.

Normal levels are tiny—under 4.0 nanograms per milliliter (ng/ml), or about 4 parts per billion. Not only is the absolute level of PSA watched, but so is the velocity with which it rises over time. A general formula is that an increase of 0.75 ng/ml over a year's time is a matter for concern, even if the absolute numbers remain in the normal range.

The PSA is the best screening method we have so far, but like most such tests it is not perfect. PSAs can miss 15 to 25 percent of prostate cancers and register a false positive result about 30 percent of the time. The false positive elevations occur from a variety of conditions, including enlargement of the gland in a condition called benign prostatic hypertrophy that develops as men age. An infected or inflamed gland, or one that has been injured, also causes PSA levels to rise. Even sexual activity can elevate PSA, which is why men are told to abstain from sex for two days before the test is performed.

Additional refinements of the PSA test help doctors further sort out PSA elevations. As noted above, the rate of rise in the PSA over time is one of them. Analyzing components of the protein in the blood is another: about 25 percent of the PSA circulating in the blood is called free, while the rest is bound to another protein. If the level of free PSA is less than 10 percent, there is a better than fifty-fifty chance that the abnormal test means cancer. (Another way doctors sometimes express this is that the ratio of free to bound PSA is lower in patients with untreated prostate cancer.)

What particularly rankles many of the PSA critics is that even with these refinements, elevated test results still trigger some unneeded procedures. And unnecessary biopsies and surgery for slow-growing tumors that might not even show up during a man's lifetime also cost money. In other words, it's the mammogram story all over again.

Though there is ongoing controversy among preventive care physicians as to whether the test is more harmful than helpful, the public airing of the limitations of PSA screening has not caused the rancor and controversy that have dogged mammograms for years. I wonder why. Is it that so many titans of industry, political leaders, generals, and other men of influence have celebrated their own brush with early and curable prostate cancer thanks to the PSA test? What politician or policy maker would dare deprive other men of their shot at early detection? Face it: until we have a better way to identify this all-too-common disease early in its course, the PSA is here to stay. It's also one number men of a certain age talk about, as they trade their PSAs as freely as they trade their blood pressure and cholesterol levels. The beauty of having a *number* is undeniable. We women are left with the vagueness of cloudy pictures.

For Everyone: Colonoscopy at Middle Age

Routine colonoscopy sets the gold standard for preventive oncology. By directly visualizing the lining of the entire large bowel, this procedure, in the hands of a skilled physician, can both detect early cancer and cure it at the same time by identifying and clipping out pre-cancerous polyps or early tumors.

Sigmoidoscopy (or proctoscopy) can be done easily in a physician's office, but it examines only the rectum and lower part of the large bowel and can miss polyps or cancers higher up. In contrast, during a colonoscopy a thin fiber-optic tube is snaked through the entire large bowel; it takes a bit longer and generally calls for mild sedation. The biggest annoyance for colonoscopy is the prep to clean out the entire colon the day before. But the good news is that if there are no polyps, the test needs to be repeated only once every seven to ten years. The exam interval is shortened to about three years or less if there is a strong family history, if pre-cancerous polyps are detected, or if the patient has a condition that predisposes to colon cancer, such as ulcerative colitis.

There's been lots of splash about the development of virtual colonoscopy using a CT scan as a way to get around the need for passing a fiber-optic tube throughout the entire bowel. It's not quite as easy as it sounds, however. A virtual study still calls for the same kind of bowel prep the day before, and the test cannot detect small polyps or clip them out at the time of detection. Current technology still requires the insertion of a rectal tube (to fill the colon with air) as well as radiation exposure. However, virtual colonoscopy is yet in its infancy and may well offer an alternative for both doctor and patient in the years ahead.

Missing from the Revolution

"Why did I do all those push-ups?" This—or some variant of it—is not an uncommon thought for those who have done it all pretty right over the years yet find themselves with a serious and advanced tumor. I certainly had those thoughts, and sometimes still do. The fact is that, however much medicine now preaches prevention and early detection, we still have no way to find some of the worst tumors before they are out of control. I think I speak for all of us when I say that medicine can and must do better.

Look at cancer of the ovary, for example. With no screening test to call its own, ovarian cancer silently spreads its malignant seeds throughout the pelvis and abdomen. Without notice, without pain, clumps of tumor attach to the lining of the body cavities, on the surface of the colon and liver, and high up under the diaphragm, weeping cancer-laden fluid that sometimes measures in the gallons. But growing deep within the pelvis, the tumor lurks without giving early signs of its presence. The same is true for other cancers that doctors have no effective way to pick up early on, including cancers of the pancreas, lung, bladder, and brain. Indeed, patients with these cancers are entirely right to wonder if the war on cancer has passed them by.

Developing effective early tests for these tumors is hardly an impossible task. A number of new blood tests are far along in development or already available. But they are proving woefully slow to appear in routine office screening among high-risk people who have no symptoms of cancer. One example is a urine test for bladder cancer that can measure levels of the matrix protein NMP22 rapidly in an office setting. (This is a tumor that is notorious for being hard to detect until it needs extensive treatment.) When NMP22 is elevated to a certain level, there is a 90 percent chance of picking up a developing bladder cancer, even when it's a small, low-grade, superficial cluster of cancerous cells. A recent analysis has also shown that in a population with a 4 percent incidence of bladder cancer—for example, heavy smokers over the age of fifty—there would be a cost savings of $100,000 or more because of less need for total bladder removal, chemotherapy, and other maintenance care. The model also showed a survival advantage of three extra years of life.

In a similar lab test for ovarian cancer, a pattern of abnormal proteins in the blood identifies those with early disease with more than a 95 percent certainty. But proponents of the test have come up against the same logic that fuels the mammogram wars, a logic that says the screening of a healthy but high-risk population with a less-than-perfect test leads to relatively large numbers of individuals with false positive results that demand further studies and, in some cases, surgical biopsies. This means anxiety for the patient and, at a societal level, a monetary cost for each tumor detected across the population that is not deemed by some policy makers as cost-effective. This calculus is useful, but if stringently applied it will slow access to universal early cancer detection. This at a time when the genomics and proteomics revolution is on the verge of making tumors discoverable early using biomarkers.

Cancers have their own genetic identity, which makes them show up in diagnostic tests for protein markers in the blood or other body fluids, and finding the right tests for these unique genetic signatures of specific tumors is the way of the future. Lance Liotta, a former NIH researcher now at George Mason University and a pioneer in the field of biomarker screening, sees the blood or other body fluids as veritable treasure troves for early cancer screening. Since these signatures mirror the genetic makeup of tumors of all types, they offer hope for detecting with a simple blood test virtually any cancer earlier rather than later.

What's keeping these new tests from doctors' offices, particularly for the cancers that have no early screening technology, is that they are being held to biological standards virtually unseen in the other screening tests widely in use today—in some cases a sensitivity and specificity requirement of over 99 percent. That is, to get to the clinic, many researchers want them to be near perfect, with an error rate of less than 1 percent. Were such perfection applied to the mammogram, the Pap smear, or PSA screening, none of them would be routinely available (or reimbursed) today. These lifesaving tests seeped into medical practice years ago, and by the trial and error of clinical studies, doctors found them to be of great value. For high-risk patients facing many of the cancers we are unable to find early, there are tests locked in the lab that are a whole lot better than the nothing we have now.

Let's recall the wisdom of the Boston cancer specialist Sidney Farber, who in the middle of the last century, long before war was declared on cancer, brought "Jimmy" to public attention. An anonymous and loveable twelve-year-old, Jimmy was an everychild, suffering with cancer at a time when there was no hope. Dr. Farber turned to the airwaves to plead for a nationally coordinated effort on Jimmy's behalf and on behalf of all those dying "this year." Though he supported research in every way, he did not believe we should wait until research satisfied some abstract notion of ideal.

Indeed, research always serves the patients of tomorrow; this is good, but we must also do the best we can for the patients of today. This includes those who face a high cancer risk or are already silently incubating cancer cells without having a means to know about it. We must relieve the future suffering of these patients now with better prevention and early cancer detection, just as we are compelled to help those with full-blown disease. The current century will be the era of cancer prevention and control—we may not achieve the historic holy grail of universal cancer cure in the twenty-first century, but that does not mean we cannot win our war.

PART FOUR

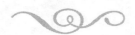

Treatment's New Era

And let thy blows, doubly redoubled,
Fall like amazing thunder on the casque
Of thy adverse pernicious enemy.

—*RICHARD II,*
WILLIAM SHAKESPEARE

CHAPTER 9

Getting Started

WHATEVER'S NEXT, IT WON'T BE PLEASANT. That thought kept repeating itself in my mind as the tumor diagnosis sank in. I knew the life detour that my family and I now faced would not be easy, and that it would be drawn out, no matter which way things broke. In fact, that was part of the reason I had chosen cardiology as my field of specialty and not oncology. Cardiovascular treatments seemed so precise, predictable, and relatively kind to the body, barely interrupting the normal scheme of things. And they were just so beautifully logical: If you have a coronary blockage that is limiting blood flow to the heart, bypass it with surgery or open it up with an angioplasty catheter and watch the blood pour through. If fluid builds up in the body, give a diuretic and in short order the lungs or legs get less congested and the urine flows. If blood clots are forming, administer a blood thinner. When cholesterol or blood pressure is too high, prescribe a few pills and measure the numbers until you get them right. The treatments are visible, their commonsense results almost immediate. That's what I wanted as a young doctor, and it's what I longed for as a patient as well: lay out the treatment, get rid of the problem, and let me be on my way, pronto.

This is not the case for most patients who face invasive cancer. The world of invisible cells is foreign to most, their reckless behavior in cancer largely inscrutable. Therapeutic choices are mindbogglingly complex, and treatments for all but the most localized of malignancies are drawn out, with uncertain results. Cancer treatment has a risk-benefit analysis all its own; the therapy is rough and toxic to an extent that seems almost to challenge the medical precept "First, do no harm." If this is going to change, it will be for one major reason: that we understand the rationale of cancer as clearly as we do the logic and mechanics of cardiovascular illness. And because cancer is a disease of genes and their proteins, we must understand their networks and interactions as well as we do the circulatory system. This is a big idea—*the* big idea, and one that is causing scientists to recast their thinking about the illness and its current and future treatments.

Fortunately, the revolution is already under way. The Human Genome Project was a boon for accelerating our knowledge about genes, the masters of cancer's fate. As a follow-up, the Cancer Genome Atlas will put the focus on cancer treatment, sketching out blueprints for the dysfunctional molecular networks that turn a cell cancerous. And sifting through the genetic and molecular profiles of individual cancers has exposed a big secret that misled many treatments of the past: that what seem to be identical tumors under the microscope can be markedly different where it really matters—in the genes and proteins. This is a crucial discovery, explaining for the first time why a tumor melts away under a particular therapy while another of the same type is barely touched, why one tumor returns in a few years yet another disappears for a lifetime. And it is a discovery that demands a rethinking of the traditional treatment approach, in which any and all cells with rapidly replicating DNA—malignant or not—are attacked as if they were known enemies of the body. The new era instead relies upon an armory of laser-like drugs, some old, some new, some yet to be devised, that specifically target deranged genetic pathways and swoop in for the kill, leaving the innocent bystanders intact—like the peregrine falcon going after its prey.

There's another, even subtler goal, which is to get ahead of the problem: to suppress a pre-cancerous clone of cells, or encourage it to differentiate toward the mature normal cell rather than devolve into a more primitive, cancerous form. If we can read the signs of future malignancy early enough, it should be possible to intervene in the life of misbehaving cells, re-forming and redirecting them before they commit to the dark side. To be sure, we are in the early phase of this new model, but the wave of change is moving fast. In my own predicament, I was lucky to find myself, in a small way, on the initial crest.

My Treatment: Old and New

The standard treatment for most brain tumors is surgery followed by radiation. In the past, chemotherapy has been considered a bust because of a natural protective wall, called the blood-brain barrier, that denies most agents floating in the blood entry into brain tissue. Specialized cells that line the brain's blood vessels create tight junctions impermeable to all but the brain's essential shopping list of small molecules such as glucose and oxygen. Larger molecules can get through, too, but only with the help of special keys in the form of carrier proteins, which grant them passage through specific channels. This barrier, so important to isolating the brain from blood-borne disease, also shields brain malignancies from many commonly used chemotherapy drugs that might otherwise destroy them. Historically, chemotherapy for brain tumors was the last-ditch "salvage therapy" when all other options had been exhausted. And sometimes, mysteriously, a tumor did respond.

From the beginning of my own journey I told my medical team that radiotherapy was not for me. Though this treatment typically makes brain tumors shrink and can lengthen life, long-term exposure to the radiation also puts patients at risk for memory and cognitive difficulties. That was one risk I chose not to take, a conviction formed more by the patient in me than from any bias I had as a physician.

Each of us owns our dreams. At that particular twist in the road, I wanted nothing more than just to be me for as long as possible—with my kids, with my husband, at home, at work. Plus, as a lifelong geek, I could not bear to threaten this brain of mine that had done me so well over the years. We were old friends, my brain and I. We were going to fight this battle together, and I would not hang on to the sort of life that came at its expense. I can't say that this is the right decision for anyone else, but it was for me.

We did not make that decision without a lot of thought. Dr. Patrick Sweeney, my neurologist and now primary care doctor, facilitated a sit-down meeting with my husband, me, and the brain trust late one afternoon about a week after surgery to discuss the final decision. Each doctor on the brain tumor team brought his own perspective. We all knew of studies showing that at least some patients with my tumor seemed to do well with chemo alone. But that was nonetheless not accepted therapy, as the clinic's radiation oncologist, Roger Macklis, stressed to us. He presented the experience with treatment of gliomas, but most were the more common glioblastoma multiforme. He also outlined the improvements in radiation therapy that have limited many of the treatment's side effects. Bruce Cohen, a pediatric neurologist, had hard-won respect for the side effects of radiation, which can be particularly evident in young children, and was sympathetic to my concern.

Dr. Gene Barnett, the surgeon and chairman of the Brain Tumor Institute, where he also conducted research on gliomas, acknowledged how little we knew about the unusual properties of my tumor, the less common oligodendroglioma, which might be more chemosensitive. From his perspective, there was no real evidence to guide us to a certain path, and good old-fashioned clinical judgment and patient choice had to weigh in heavily. David Peereboom, the neuro-oncologist who would be providing the treatments, was comfortable delaying radiation if the tumor proved sensitive to drugs. He optimistically pointed out that small blood vessels can be scarred by radiation and make chemo's entry even more of a problem, singling out this approach as a sensible one, at least in theory. And he did not flinch at the thought that other oncologists might see this as lesser care; it was ultimately an informed patient's choice.

Brian Bolwell came at this from his experience with tumors of the blood and bone marrow. Never wilting from challenging established dogma, he supported Fred's and my decision all the way. (Only later did I learn that he was one of a small group of top oncologists who were leading the emerging practice of avoiding, if possible, chest radiation in young Hodgkin's patients because of late-onset complications of heart scarring and breast cancer.) He reminded me that so much of cancer treatment is trial and error, and it's common to change the script midway into the run, substituting one therapy for another based on an individual's choice, unexpected complications, and tumor response. My brain trust would often say, "Cancer therapies will never be chiseled in stone, Bernie." And this was not a garden-variety tumor with a lot of strong science behind it anyway. So I had my docs behind me and we had our plan: surgery, chemo, then patience.

A certain relief comes once the battle plan is laid out. Preparations for treatment then take over, and you move on mind-numbed autopilot—a respite from the early rush of emotions propelled by the uneasy feeling of being lost in a strange and unkind land. The Taussig Cancer Center became my new home. A decade before, when I was head of the Research Institute at the Cleveland Clinic, my office was on the large corridor leading to the cancer center. In those days, I saw many patients come and go in various stages of therapy and felt so sorry for their plight. During that time,

I launched two new research departments at the Clinic, one in molecular biology and genetics, the other in cancer biology. Who would have thought that I would be walking down that same corridor years later, only as a patient, having my brain tissue studied in the clinic's research labs, and wondering what blessings tomorrow's science might bring as a result.

I was fast becoming a professional patient, guided by a daily schedule of clinic and hospital stops that left little time for much else. During one appointment, I met with the nurse practitioners at the Brain Tumor Institute and saw Dr. Barnett to have my head staples removed; on another I had a post-op MRI. Then there were two more visits to the operating room to have special catheters installed through tiny incisions beneath my collarbones. Blood tests, mostly to monitor assorted blood counts, were regular events. My poor arms began to show the telltale needle marks and bruises of my patienthood.

I became somewhat uncomfortable when I realized how much time this was taking. I had other things to do: a briefcase full of work, a ton of phone calls, and two big conference calls about the newly created Public Health School that was in the process of becoming nationally accredited at Ohio State—the first in the state. And, just one week before I fell ill, my husband and I had signed a contract for a second home in Florida, thinking that someday we might want to join the flock of Cleveland snowbirds escaping the cold winter months. I was in charge of that transaction and of getting us settled in over spring break, which was coming up in just three weeks. We were taking Marie and a few of her friends with us, and at that juncture there was nothing more I wanted to do. On top of this we had to do our taxes, something that knows no excuses. This tumor stuff really had come at a most inconvenient time.

I also had to get myself ready for the possibility of bone marrow transplantation. Chemotherapy drugs attack the replicating DNA of rapidly growing cancer cells. Because stem cells, too, grow and divide quickly in order to produce the ever refreshed white and red blood cells that circulate in our bloodstream, they are a primary victim of chemo's collateral damage. Some drugs are particularly likely to wipe out the bone marrow. Since there was a promising experimental drug that was just being tested in patients whose tumors had failed radiation therapy (which my doctors thought might be an option if the first choice of chemo drugs bombed), we had to be ready. Thus, I had to bank healthy bone marrow stem cells before they got a whiff of the toxic chemo agents that could damage them.

The stem cell collection process—called apheresis, after the Greek word meaning "to take away"—involved sifting the cells out of my blood and then tucking them away in a freezer where they would be safe and sound for at least ten years. Harvesting stem cells is actually a bigger deal than one might imagine. Central to stem cell collection is a novel device, the Hickman catheter. These spaghetti-sized tubes are threaded through the veins that run under the clavicle, ending up in the deep venous system near the heart. The catheters allow large volumes of blood to flow in and out of the body as it passes through a cell-sorting machine, which is designed to pluck out just the tiny stem cells and collect them in a plastic bag, a little like an old-time prospector sifting river sand for nuggets of gold.

As a cardiologist, I was quite familiar with central venous lines. They are standard equipment in cardiac care units, where, hooked up to gauges, they measure blood pressure within the veins, a surrogate measure of blood volume and heart function. They also provide secure access to a patient's bloodstream to draw blood and administer needed drugs, and for that reason central catheters came to be used for cancer patients. The Hickman is a portable version of the central line. They offer the hookup lines to the apheresis machine to pull off stem cells for bone marrow transplants, and they also are the portal for delivering lifesaving stem cells into patients who are undergoing bone marrow transplants.

After brain surgery, this procedure was a cakewalk. Dr. Michael Geisinger had done tons of them. And the anesthesiologist, Walter

Maurer, a colleague at the Clinic for years, was a comforting friend—and not just because of the intravenous Versed that kept me in a vague twilight zone. I knew what was happening but deliciously floated along without a care in the world—until I was abruptly returned to earth once the tubes were in. Then I was faced with yet another task, that of hiding two bulky tubes coiled under a white gauze bandage beneath my blouse.

Not long ago I had a good laugh with a dear friend and fellow cancer survivor, Dr. Victor Fazio. Vic is a world-renowned leader in colorectal surgery at the Cleveland Clinic, with plenty of dealings with cancer patients. But he had his own personal experience with Hickman catheters during a bone marrow transplant for a bout with leukemia a few years previously. As he put it in his delightful Aussie accent, "I had no idea how much was involved here. I used to order these things like I was ordering grapes." Indeed, these catheters are uneasy houseguests in the body, requiring lots of tender care. Among other things, the tubes must be flushed with an injection of heparin every day to keep them from clotting up with blood. I was fortunate in that my husband took on this responsibility, even though it was not an easy thing for him to do as his final chore before going off to work at 6 A.M. Fred did a good job of bucking up my spirits by regarding me as if I were quite well, and I knew that confronting the contrary evidence by caring for the catheters and periodically drawing blood at the kitchen table was a hard chore for him emotionally. Surgeons don't operate on their loved ones, and though this was not exactly heart surgery, tending the bandages of his wounded wife cast him visibly into the awkward role of being both doctor and husband.

Stem cell collection also relies on a clever drug innovation to juice up production of the marrow's stem cells. Normally, stem cells live and grow in the bone marrow but are scarce in the bloodstream. For stem cells to be efficiently gathered from the blood their numbers must first be increased, or it would take forever to collect the millions of them that are needed for a transplant. Daily injections of a bioengineered medicine called Neupogen (or G-CSF, short for granulocyte-colony stimulating factor) do just that. It drives the bone marrow to produce white cells and their parent stem cells at bulging levels, which then spill out into the blood. After a few daily self-injections (something most patients can learn to do), you know the drug is working—your bones start to throb, particularly the breastbone and pelvis, due to the sudden swelling of marrow mass within a very limited bone-encased space. After six days of Neupogen, a quadrupling of my normal white blood cell count, and some pretty achy bones, I was ready to be "sorted out."

The goal was to harvest 9 million stem cells over several days. It was a painless process conducted by Anna Koo, who had done research on apheresis during the years I headed the Research Institute. I was pleasantly surprised to see her smiling face, but at the same time the surprise brought home how hard it was for a doctor being cared for in her own hospital to hide anonymously under a scarf or behind a book—which is just what I wanted to do at that point. Illness is a private time; however kind those around you may be, sometimes you just want to crawl off into a corner and not have to face anyone until it's all over.

All went well—until there were about 6.5 million stem cells in the apheresis bag. At that point, the number of platelets in my blood began to fall precipitously. I knew something was up when Dr. Bolwell appeared unexpectedly and with a furrowed brow said he had enough stem cells and to stop the collection. Because of the platelets' small size they can be sifted out, too, and if too many are extracted, there is a risk of uncontrolled bleeding. I knew we had not quite reached the initial goal, so I urged Dr. Bolwell to continue on—patients can do just fine with modestly low platelets. But on this he would not bend. He had enough cells to do a transplant, he said, and because I had just had neurosurgery there was an increased risk of bleeding. Dr. Barnett was in full agreement, and Dr. Bolwell not only stopped the collection but ordered a platelet transfusion as well.

Despite my subsequent life as head of the American Red Cross, I've never been keen on blood transfusions. Rather, I should say, I have profound respect for their risks. I always preached to my students not to take them lightly—that any patient who had a one-unit transfusion has had one too many, for patients can almost always tolerate a one-unit blood loss and can easily recover in a short period of time with some iron pills. Transfusions should be used only if there is a big need—two or more units. Dr. Bolwell reminded me, however, that to get my platelets up I needed a "five-pack," that is, a pool of platelets taken from five units of blood. So I lost that one, too, and went ahead with what was to be the first of several transfusions over the next several months. I had given blood many times, going back to my years in medical school when the donation habit started. (Truth time: in those days we also got paid $25, which did encourage penniless med students to extend their arms.) But this was going to be the first time I would receive a transfusion. In my book, only sick people got them. And part of my resistance, no doubt, was that I didn't want to face yet another measure that I was, by some standards, sick.

When I got home, still woozy from the intravenous Benadryl given to ward off an allergic reaction to the transfusion, I climbed into our cozy bed, finished the last few pages of my book, and fell into soothing sleep. When I awoke Mom was there, just checking on me, as she would say; it was as if I were her little girl again. She had raised four daughters, lost a husband nearly twenty years before, and now at seventy-seven years of age was tending to me, the daughter who was supposed to be looking after her. Mom always rallied when things were tough. She and my sister Michele, my junior by eleven months but now very much the stronger one, kept up with my daily treatment chronicles, but they also kept my unexpected detour in proper proportion by always finding something we could all laugh about.

Michele would remind me with her mischievous smile that I was not the only person having a rough time. Look, for example, at

Monica Lewinsky and Bill Clinton, who were big items in the news then; look at what their families were facing. Our talk at dinner that night quickly shifted from my stem cells to whether our dear ninety-eight-year-old Nonie, who we all saw as a perfectly proper Victorian lady, was going to watch the heavily touted Lewinsky interview to be aired on TV later that night. Probably so, Nonie said, and Mom, Missy, and I agreed to join her. Fred thought it was all nonsense, and Marie, fortunately, had homework to do. Life went on, and I forgot for a while that a day later I had another trip back to the Clinic to deal with my bulky Hickman catheters.

The Hickman would do double duty. After the stem cell harvest, I was back in the operating room with Drs. Geisinger and Maurer to remove one catheter and convert the other into a permanent venous port. The conversion involves placing a small button-shaped device under the skin attached to the end of the indwelling catheter. In the center of the button is a diaphragm that can be pierced by a needle—just as a vein in your arm is—to get access to the bloodstream. It becomes a portal for administering chemotherapy, and for giving or drawing blood. Chemo drugs are especially rough on the small, relatively fragile veins in the arms, making them scar and over time turn into knotty, fibrous cords impossible to be tapped for blood. By injecting the sclerosing drugs directly into the port, the veins of the arms are spared, and the chemo is diluted in the large central veins, where it does no damage. As alien as it may seem, I grew oddly fond of this new addition to my body perched just beneath my left clavicle and just above my heart. Perhaps it was because the port was a symbol of how new technology was protecting the innocent tissues that would otherwise be blitzed by chemo's collateral damage. Or maybe it was more primal than that: this tiny Purple Heart hidden beneath my clothes marked a difficult time that I was planning to survive.

But I had little time to admire it. Barely a day after the Hickman became a port I met with Dr. Peereboom, who loaded me down with a brown bag filled with carefully marked vials of pills. Oncologists are fond of administering cocktails, coded by the first initial of the name of each drug; my cocktail code was PCV, for procarbazine and CCNU (also known as lomustine), to be taken orally, and vincristine, to be administered through the port. Dr. Peereboom's oncology nurse, Mary Miller, handed me a calendar that laid out the complicated four-week cycle, indicating the days to begin and end each medicine, along with the times to get my blood drawn. Also marked week by week were the dates when I might expect my blood counts to begin dropping. Chemo drugs have a way of going after the bone marrow, but just how much varies from patient to patient and drug to drug. The calendar also marked the time for my next MRI. That would tell us just how sensitive the beast inside would be to the chemical onslaught, and guide further therapy. In this first cycle of chemo there were no promises, only hope.

Still, hope does soften the side effects—which quickly came to mind when I saw the accompanying prescriptions for anti-nausea medicines. There was one for the widely used Compazine, and another for a newer drug, Kytril, more powerful but more expensive, at $50 per pill. I thought I would start using the cheaper pills and turn to the expensive stuff only if I really needed it. I also knew a lot about Compazine: it was time-tested, a drug I had administered to many of my own patients over the years. My general philosophy about medicines is to move to the new agents only if you have a good reason to.

Chemo starts easy, with few side effects. On day one of the first week of treatment I took lomustine and felt great. A good thing, since that same week I had to go back to the wig lady to pick up my newly crafted hair, a surprisingly weird experience. Sitting in what looked like a very small but private beauty salon in her shop, I neither felt like a beauty nor wanted to have my hair done. I watched with quiet detachment as Carolyn and her assistant, John, put the thing on my head and started clipping, trying to match my own tresses. Mine were by no means as lush as their creation, but still, I liked them better. This new mop was clearly someone else's. Carolyn and John chatted away as hairdressers commonly do, telling me how I was one of their calmest clients facing this ordeal. I guess I was just better at not showing how unnerved I really was. Fortunately, Fred was there with me, quietly reading in a chair nearby. Besides, we had a dinner to go to after this with some prominent people who were doing some good things for the Clinic, so I had no choice but to keep it together.

This experience was part of steeling myself for the many side effects of chemo that have become so deeply chiseled into cancer folklore. I was no exception. My appetite dropped like a rock, along with my weight, calling into action those out-of-fashion skinny clothes I should have tossed years before but had instead stuffed away in the attic. The warm ones, that is, since I always seemed to be cold. Food tastes changed—everything I put into my mouth tasted metallic—and my skin dried up like a broken twig. Doctors tell you how important exercise routines are in cancer care, but the best intentions run up against visibly vanishing muscles and often lose the standoff. As for my hair, about half of it did fall out. I thought I disguised this famously with some heavy-duty hair spray that seemed to double the thickness of the surviving strands—and could probably have frozen a bird in flight. Occasionally I donned my trusty wig, but I never did really figure out how to keep the darn thing straight.

My first blast of chemo's toxicity came during the second week of this initial chemo cycle. On day eight I started the P in PCV, procarbazine pills, for a two-week daily stint. Also on that day I had my first dose of vincristine, the V of the triple cocktail. As the plan went, I would have a second dose of vincristine on day twenty-nine to complete the first cycle of chemo, and two weeks later I'd start the whole cycle again.

Unlike the other drugs that I could take in the comfort of home, vincristine required an in-person appearance at one of the treatment rooms on the first floor of the cancer center. From a recliner—generally known as the chemo chair—I watched the ritual of my first encounter with vincristine unfold. Who would think that the lovely periwinkle plant with its polished dark green leaves and blue and purple flowers could be the natural source of such a fearsome drug, which not only tears into cancer but, as a descendant of mustard gas, is also a blistering agent that damages tissue on contact and is treated with great respect by its handlers? After all, it was the reason for my newly placed port, which Maureen Bell, my sunny and cheerful oncology nurse, was getting ready to test for the first time. She laid out the necessary paraphernalia, including an intravenous setup that was hooked up to the newly placed port. Dr. Geisinger was there to check his handiwork on its first occasion of use to be sure the catheter was not clogged or kinked. We all held our breath for a moment as Maureen pulled back on the syringe she had attached to the port and attempted to draw back blood. She pulled effortlessly as the red stuff flowed, and everyone seemed to smile at once. The port worked perfectly—a little victory. Dr. Sweeney did a quick neurological exam—peered into the back of my eyes with an ophthalmoscope and checked a few reflexes—and I was ready. As the vincristine dripped in, Dr. Peereboom dropped by for a few words of encouragement, Dr. Cohen came over to review my chart, and Dr. Bolwell stuck his head in to say something like, "You have too many doctors here, and by the way, are you exercising?"

He was possibly right about the doctors, but it was one of the quiet comforts of being in a place where your friends of many years are caring for you. The real benefit, however, and one available to all patients at Taussig and many other cancer centers, is that I was in a place where my doctors worked side by side, sharing the same corridors and treatment rooms, interacting easily with each other, and coming together for only one reason: to care for someone in distress. But I had no such philosophical musings at that moment; I just kept my eyes on the vincristine, realizing the nasty stuff was being delivered straight to my heart. It was puzzling to me that, of the three drugs in my cocktail, this was the one least likely to get by the blood-brain barrier. Why, then, was it still being used? I rhetorically posed that question to my docs, but the answer boils down to: just because. Because that's what seems to work sometimes. Maybe it's not targeted medicine, but that's all there was.

Whatever its value would be, I was initiated into the world of chemotherapy; I'd been touched by all three drugs. And it didn't seem too bad—until later that night, when I discovered what made chemo so darkly famous. A little after midnight, nausea, dry heaves, and vomiting hit suddenly, and recurred like clockwork every forty-five minutes. Exhausted, I would fall asleep as each wave passed, but unfairly so, as my husband, who had a job to go to in the morning, was awake all night. This happened for several nights in a row, as if my body was primitively and relentlessly reacting to the toxic stuff seeping into it by its rhythmic calls of rejection, a protective mechanism no doubt programmed into our genes over the ages. Dr. Peereboom mentioned that procarbazine was most apt to be the culprit, but the procarbazine-vincristine combination was more troublesome on this score than either drug alone. I wondered if that stomach misery might mean that vincristine was actually making it up to my brain after all. Somewhere in my lexicon of medical facts I recalled that the brain had a chemoreceptor trigger zone to signal the nearby vomiting center if something was afoul.

These musings made me feel only a tad better, and so I vowed to take the heavy-duty anti-nausea medicine in all future cycles. After that, queasy was the worst of it—and I have never been so grateful for queasy. I've come away from this experience appreciating just how awful chemo must have been before the discovery of the more powerful anti-nausea medicines. As quality-of-life meds, they don't get much attention, and might even be written off as nonessential. To the contrary. These new drugs gave me, as they give many, a semblance of normalcy during a long stretch of toxic treatment.

But there was something else that helped me get through this medical *annus horribilis*. Four days before I began chemo, I heard some news about my tumor. I was at home and had just finished listening to a guided imagery tape with a mellifluous voice telling me I was on a warm sandy beach with the waves gently lapping around me. It just didn't work, at least not on that icy Cleveland day. I did better focusing on the medical school, so I spent the rest of the morning with Brenda Hammond and Sara Strong. They were my pals, and my trusted assistants in the dean's office at Ohio State. Together they managed to keep things flowing back and forth from Columbus to Cleveland throughout my early treatment, and always with a good joke or some juicy news to lighten things up. That day, Brenda and I were discussing an overdue essay I had promised to write for *Time* magazine, about Ian Wilmut and the implications of his cloned sheep Dolly. It was scheduled to appear in a special science and medicine issue in late March. Out of sheer necessity, Brenda was for the first time introducing me to the great world of e-mail, which was the only way for me to get it to the editors by their deadline. I'd also just received a lovely note from the head of the Ohio State dental school, Henry Fields, echoing Brenda's optimism that I'd be back at the medical school soon. To be precise, I was planning to return full time by match day, March 18, just ten days away. Match day is an annual rite of spring in medical education, when the graduating students find out all at once where they will spend their next several years in residency. I wanted the answer, too; what did the future hold for me? With more confidence than I felt, I assured Brenda that I'd be there.

Just then my husband called with news from my surgeon, Dr. Barnett. Part of the gene analysis was in, and my tumor matched the profile of those in the Toronto study that responded well to chemotherapy. Like mine, those tumors were all missing the short arm of chromosome 1. So there was a good chance that my tumor would be chemosensitive, too. My husband and I both choked up. Though we were still awaiting the results of other gene tests, this one broken chromosome was a good omen and reason for cautious hope. There was now a very good chance that the nasty clump of cells putting me in this fix was in for trouble.

How odd that a mangled chromosome was music to my ears. A concept entirely alien to me a few weeks before now looked like my ticket to return to work, maybe to see my girls' next graduations, to have some of those brief vacations with Fred that in the past had seemed so difficult to squeeze into our schedules. I knew this field of cancer genetics was still in its infancy and that I should not overreact, but learning about chromosome 1, and then a few weeks later that it had a partner in arm deletion on chromosome 19 (another characteristic of the brain tumors analyzed in the Canadian study), gave me a logical reason for believing that I might have a chance. I was lucky, when of course luck is a relative thing. Having this gene profile—even though our optimism was based on a still-early finding in a handful of patients—seemed just then to make up for any prayers that had gone unanswered in the past.

As I latched on to these nanobits of gene information, I wondered how it would have been had I gotten the opposite news. I would still want to know, I decided, but why, when it would only be a downer? I guess because I was already in that mode; I was already steeled for getting less favorable news, which I think is common when people first confront a cancer diagnosis. Only a few days before, I'd found myself quietly looking for my old copy of Elisabeth Kübler-Ross's *On Death and Dying*—a classic text, but not one of my favorites even when I was first introduced to it in my early medical training. Perhaps a less positive gene reading would have influenced how I spent my time, or increased my resolve to move sooner to more aggressive, experimental chemo with a bone marrow transplant by summer. Maybe I would have opted for a lighter work schedule. But then again, maybe not—kicking back wasn't appealing under any circumstances, least of all the current ones. My family had to carry on with their lives, and I drew strength from knowing that I had to do the same.

As time went by, more information on my tumor genes trickled in. In my genetic musings, I began to focus not only on the two mangled chromosomes but also on the apparent health of my copies of $p53$, a gene that, as I've mentioned, functions as a guardian of the genome, a master at triggering bad cells to quietly do themselves

in—that is, to undergo apoptosis when their genes become hope-
lessly deranged. I could just see my tumor's mangled chromosomes
being further damaged by the drugs that were about to soak my
body. I could imagine the distorted DNA prompting $p53$ to signal a
stern suicide order. It seemed like an easy and logical kill, not calling
on too much fancy work. Logical and rational—and surely simplis-
tic. But that's okay. These musings became my own special version
of guided imagery. I'd just close my eyes and watch those tired-out,
ugly cells drop off one by one, like the leaves of a tree in autumn.

CHAPTER 10

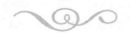

Why Cancer Treatment Works

IT IS NOT THE leaves of autumn that permeate most thinking about cancer treatment. Rather, it's the rough imagery of war, both at a macro level in the national fight to find a cure and more intimately in the battles of the individual cancer patient. Cancer treatment is tough stuff, and its well-earned reputation is very much a part of the big chill that comes with a cancer diagnosis. To be sure, conventional cancer therapy is a kind of military assault on the rapidly proliferating cells that are trying to take over: it cuts the alien clones out with a scalpel, hits the tumor zone locally with a radiation attack, and infuses chemicals to poison roaming cancer cells that have escaped from the tumor bed. In this scenario, the weapons of the cancer war subject the body as innocent bystander to substantial collateral damage.

For all this, the success of cancer treatment is more elegant than we ever imagined. As we probe the malignant cell and study its molecular behavior, a strange logic comes into view. We see that radiation and chemotherapy work because they use the body's own defenses to rid itself of cancer. Unbeknownst to the physicians who pioneered these strategies half a century ago, part of their effectiveness comes from the natural process of apoptosis, forcing useless or dangerous cells to self-destruct. This process is central to health, as it prunes unneeded cells and sloughs aged ones—and destroys the botched cancer cells quietly, invisibly, and often before we even know they are there. In cancer treatment, the radiation and chemotherapy injure the cancer cells just enough to trigger this biological phenomenon, explaining how tumors can visibly shrink with each cycle of chemotherapy or radiation exposure, and do so without bleeding, inflammation, or pain. The bad cells melt away like the spring snow. It could not be a better fairy-tale ending for the cancer demon.

The delicate balance maintained by apoptosis, which awesomely keeps the net number of cells in our body constant, is the secret of cancer treatment. Chemotherapy and radiation wreak their havoc on actively replicating DNA, and because cancer cells are growing rapidly, they are more likely to be taken out than are stable, healthy cells whose DNA is quiet and safely coiled up. The damage triggers a cascade of molecular signals, which under the best of circumstances spark the internal suicide switch programmed into cells' genes. Despite its many aggressive properties, the cancer genome is in fact rather fragile, its unstable, ever-mutating DNA more easily damaged than that in normal cells. The same toxins do less damage to the more disciplined DNA of healthy cells—even the frequently dividing ones in the bone marrow or gut—which explains why the body almost always recovers from even the harshest of cancer treatments.

There are other factors that stimulate the suicide program and feed into cancer-killing strategies. Some cancer cells, oxygen-starved from a rapidly growing tumor that has outgrown its blood supply, self-destruct. So, too, will those unable to produce sufficient levels of survival proteins, such as BCL-2, that keep the cell's suicide program under wraps. White blood cells that often move into a tumor can create a hostile environment by secreting a chemical called tumor necrosis factor. TNF latches on to bad-looking cells and takes them out, again by flipping on their internal suicide switches. While the surgeon uses a scalpel to remove bulky visible tumors, the body's own molecular blades destroy cells one by one, targeting them with the precision of a falcon in pursuit of its prey, while leaving healthy cells untouched. It's the peregrine's way.

Cancer is a clever demon, however, and its rapidly mutating cells fight back by knocking out the protective tumor suppressor genes or finding ways to build up their own survival proteins to drown out suicide signals. As I've mentioned, cancer cells also can produce their own heat shock proteins to protect the very molecules that drive the cells' malignant ways. They also co-opt angiogenesis, sprouting their own blood vessels to avoid strangulation from the lack of oxygen or the buildup of toxic waste products. And because they are traitors, rather than true invaders, cancer cells often retain enough of their original identities to slip through the immune system's dragnet, tricking the body into believing they are the right stuff and are not to be destroyed by roving white blood cells as other invaders would be.

This highlights a nagging problem for all cancer treatments. Cancer's genetic instability makes it vulnerable in some cases, but it also allows multiplying cells to mutate rapidly under the onslaught of chemicals or radiation, causing a once-sensitive tumor to become resistant. These mutated cancer cells once again hijack normal cell survival mechanisms, using them to pump toxic chemo drugs right back out again, or in some other manner engineer their way around previously winning therapies. That's another reason why chemotherapy is so often delivered in multidrug cocktails. The goal is to cut off cells that become resistant to one drug by giving another at the same time. However disordered cancer cells look under the microscope, they are rational in their own survivalist design.

Revolutionary Therapy

Targeted therapy aims to meet cancer's twisted molecular logic with an equally rational strategy of containment and annihilation. It is an entirely new approach to fighting cancer, by directly countering the cancer's own crafty genetic reengineering. A tumor's genetic and molecular profile tells the story of its handiwork, and one of the biggest surprises of modern cancer research is just how staggeringly complex that handiwork is—comprising not one or two genes gone wrong but a patchwork of genes that varies mightily even among seemingly identical tumors.

"Targeted therapy" is, in fact, an overly bland name for a revolutionary approach that is vastly different from the treatments patients have traditionally experienced. It's the difference between heading into hostile territory blindfolded and alone versus navigating with the benefit of maps, reconnaissance reports, and night vision goggles. Most current therapy is based not on reliable scouting reports but on a collection of observations of what happened to a group of tumors carrying the same name in which treatment results are averaged together. The resulting averages often obscure a wide standard deviation in results: some people benefit greatly, while others see no benefit, some are even harmed, and the many in between experience only a trivial difference. This is unlike most other forms of illness—from high blood pressure to blocked coronary arteries to hypothyroidism—where treatment response is almost always what's been expected. Not so for cancer.

For most of the war on cancer—some thirty-five years and counting—we didn't have the means to map and characterize individual genes and understand their function. But now, armed as we are with the knowledge and rapid and relatively inexpensive technology born of the Human Genome Project, we have no excuse not to mine this molecular treasure trove of genes and their proteins. Genetic microarrays or gene chips—ingenious devices that command a laboratory's worth of analytical power, all on a single silicon chip smaller than a postage stamp—can identify individual genes and gene expression patterns from a speck of tissue or a drop of blood, quickly and cheaply. The Cancer Genome Atlas, the newly initiated NIH project aimed at decoding the genetic behavior of the 200 most common cancers, will help guide individual cancer therapy. It may be a simple analogy, but I believe that caring for patients without this knowledge is the equivalent of a doctor pumping powerful drugs into patients with hypertension without the benefit of blood pressure readings, or a heart surgeon operating on a patient's blocked coronary arteries without the guidance of a coronary angiogram.

The analysis of my tumor for broken chromosomes was but a tiny, early step toward gene-directed care—a pilot, if you will. I can only imagine how many more secrets are still hidden in my own tumor and everyone else's. What we are learning about the vast and complex processes that enable any given nest of cancer cells to take hold and then transform to the most aggressive state of distant metastasis is good cause to ignite a new and reinvigorated war on cancer.

New Drugs

The proof of this approach is already here. Genetic knowledge has led to a slew of new drugs—some still in the research pipelines, others already in use—that are designed specifically to target a given gene or its protein product. Take, for example, the family of proteins called tyrosine kinases, which I touched on in Chapter 4. These act as on-off switches, directing many of the core cell functions such as growth, development, and survival—and cancers use them to grow and prosper. There are fifty or more varieties of these kinases, the protein products of mutated genes that turn oncogenic and contribute to specific cancers. They make an obvious target for a counterattack strategy, since blocking the initial kinase signal with a designer molecule will shut down the growth or survival pathway that follows.

One of the earliest and most successful examples of this strategy is the breast cancer drug Herceptin (trastuzumab), which was specifically designed by scientists at Genentech to block kinase receptors produced by the *HER2/neu* oncogene. These receptors lather the surface of breast cancer cells in about 30 percent of patients. The effect of this targeted drug has been palpable: before Herceptin, the news of *HER2/neu's* aggressive presence was devastating, but now this same intelligence offers more than hope. For patients diagnosed with this particular oncogene, Herceptin treatment reduces breast cancer recurrence by 50 percent after three years, and mortality by a third.

The drug Tarceva (erlotinib) targets another tyrosine kinase in the epidermal growth factor receptor (EGFR) family, which is overproduced in some cancers of the colon, prostate, brain, and lung. Like Herceptin, Tarceva benefits only patients whose tumors rely on EGFR to progress. In the case of lung cancer, that subset amounts to about 10 percent of lung cancer patients. When these patients are treated with Tarceva, their survival goes on average from one year to two. Pessimists might claim that only 10 percent of patients are helped; optimists might note that survival is doubled for the group helped.

We had better forget about the fevered search for a single silver bullet to cure all cancer; it does not exist. What these early successes show vividly is that a new era of drug discovery is here. And for this kind of work, the hit-or-miss, blind-luck approach of traditional drug development is no longer enough. The so-called rational drug design strategy, pioneered more than fifty years ago by two scientists, George Hitchings and Gertrude Elion at Burroughs Wellcome (now GlaxoSmithKline), starts with a comparison of the chemical makeup of normal and diseased cells and then exploits the differences to design drugs. Hitchings and Elion had limited technology to explore the chemical soup that makes a life, but their strategy transformed much of drug discovery, and led to a Nobel Prize for both in 1988.

Gleevec (imatinib) is another kinase inhibitor success story based on rational drug design. From the outset, scientists at Novartis sought a molecule to interrupt the action of a cancer-promoting protein produced by the Philadelphia chromosome (see Chapter 3). This chromosome, the hybrid result of the accidental swapping of parts of chromosomes 9 and 22, produces an overactive tyrosine kinase called BCR-ABL, which is present in most forms of chronic myelogenous leukemia. Hematologists have known about the Philadelphia chromosome since 1960, when physician Peter Nowell proposed that it somehow caused the blood cancer rather than being a result of it, as was then commonly thought. Almost half a century later, his discovery, amplified by knowledge of the specific genes and proteins involved, turned into a powerful new drug that induces remarkable remissions in advanced stages of leukemia.

The Gleevec story illustrates another important point: a rare cancer, a sarcoma of the stomach and small intestine called GIST—short for gastrointestinal stromal tumor—also responds to the drug. That's because Gleevec blocks another oncogene, called *c-kit* (also present in chronic myelogenous leukemia), which is a key genetic driver of GIST. This new drug has radically changed the lives of many of the 500 to 1,000 people facing this tumor each year, for whom there was no effective chemotherapy. But in a broader sense, this happy link between a leukemia and a stomach cancer validates the very notion of targeted cancer treatment: if two very different tumors carry a common gene abnormality, there is a good chance that a drug that targets that trait will work for both. This is the landmark thinking that will rewrite the practice of oncology.

But Gleevec also illustrates a problem, one that haunts most other chemotherapies: in a relentless cat-and-mouse game, malignant cells resistant to Gleevec's powers sometimes emerge from the tumor's ashes. This reinforces the strategy of using drug cocktails to attack multiple pathways and molecular sites at the same time, dealing a series of fatal blows before the tumor has time to heal its wounds and reemerge. And to keep ahead of the mutating cancer cells, two new Gleevec-like drugs—Tasigna (nilotinib) and Sprycel (dasatinib)—have been developed for patients who become resistant to Gleevec.

Still, the dramatic success of these few targeted drugs shows what this powerful strategy will someday mean for all patients. If by blocking just one on-off switch in 10 percent of patients with lung cancer, the drug Tarceva doubles their survival, imagine what we could do if we could identify all the factors contributing to the growth or spread of any given cancer. With an individual tumor's full genomic map before us, we could identify the specific cancer-promoting molecules supporting the malignancy and then prescribe a personal and specifically targeted mix of drugs. This is personalized medicine.

Another new world of drugs, most yet to be discovered or designed, will also target the on-off switches of cancer processes that work outside the cancer cell. We know that a tumor sprouts its own blood supply; Judah Folkman's dream that molecules could be developed to choke off the tumor's supply chain was realized in 2004 with Genentech's release of the anti-angiogenesis drug Avastin (bevacizumab). Designed to inhibit vascular endothelial growth factor (VEGF), which is produced in abundance in tumors on the march, Avastin slows tumor growth in advanced colon and lung cancers, with at least some marginal survival benefit. The giant has not yet fallen, but Goliath, for the first time, is starting to stumble.

Other drugs are being designed to target different components of the external matrix in which the cancer cell grows and spreads. As yet, we have limited knowledge of the gene patterns that convert local cancer cells into reckless migrants, but roving cells that create metastases have a gene mix different from many of the homebody cells they leave behind in the primary tumor. For example, if the tumor suppressor gene *PTEN* is deleted, cancer cells become more mobile. Other genes help cancer cells take root in distant organs, such as a prostate cancer cell learning to thrive in the liver. These new powers—to move, grow new blood vessels, and live next to cells that are not their type—are the result of gene reprogramming. This nasty bit of molecular contracting is waiting for the development of tailored drugs: drugs to inhibit the proteins that start the process; drugs to dull the invading cells' chemical drills as they cut through blood vessels and solid organs; drugs to block their magnetic draw to distant organs. All of these are possible and all are on the drawing board.

Some of these new cancer-fighting drugs are actually old ones. Take thalidomide, a tranquilizing and anti-nausea drug made infamous by causing birth defects back in the 1950s. As it happens, the very mechanism that interrupted blood vessel growth to stunt limb development in the fetus also stunts the growth of multiple myeloma, the bone marrow cancer. The notorious drug was still on the market, approved by the FDA for treating the rare bacterial disease leprosy, and physican researchers discovered its value in the treatment of multiple myeloma. Based on what is called "off label use," thalidomide quickly moved into mainstream cancer medicine. Cancer therapeutics often depend on such off-label administration of drugs. Since the medications are already FDA approved for other uses, physicians can prescribe them based on new or existing evidence of benefit.

Another new anti-cancer strategy focuses on controlling inflammation and other immune responses. We know that tumors spread by commandeering the body's inflammatory pathways to help them invade locally and infiltrate distant organs. For example, the cyclooxygenase-2 or COX-2 molecule, which fosters inflammation, is overactive in some cancers. If a particular tumor shows overproduction of the COX-2 protein, some oncologists consider adding anti-inflammatory agents ranging from aspirin to the more specific COX-2 inhibitors such as Celebrex to a chemo cocktail. Similarly, the body's immune system naturally produces special proteins that fight off infections. With names such as interleukin-2 and interferon, these molecules have already proven beneficial in treating certain solid tumors, including kidney cancer and blood malignancies such as leukemia and myeloma.

The effectiveness of these immune molecules in some cancers fuels the long-held dream of teaching the body's own immune defenses to target cancer cells. Cancer researcher Steven Rosenberg of the National Cancer Institute and others have devoted many years to this approach, with enough success in some patients to keep the work very much alive. Dramatic benefits have been observed in a small subset of patients with advanced forms of malignant melanoma and kidney cancer. Most recently Rosenberg has created a vaccine from melanoma patients' own white blood cells by genetically engineering the cells in the lab to become melanoma fighters and then reinfusing them back into the bloodstream, with impressive benefits to some patients with advanced disease.

A tumor vaccine—which, like all immunizations, trains the immune system to recognize and destroy an invader—also shows promise for prostate and pancreatic cancer. And vaccines that target the heat shock proteins that some tumors use to survive are also under study. On paper at least, there is no reason why we should not be able to make these and other vaccines target the unique protein patterns specific to cancer, without inciting an immune attack on normal cells. Hope continues that immunotherapy will be able to take out primary tumors as well as metastases.

Time-Honored Cancer Treatments

Exploration into the deeper mechanisms of cancer has not toppled the time-honored pillars of cancer care—surgery, chemotherapy, radiation, and bone marrow transplantation. Rather, modern molecular discoveries have validated their fundamental strategies—and also helped oncologists to use them more precisely.

Whatever treatment you face today, and however long it's been in use, you are not likely to relive your parent's or your best friend's cancer experience. So much of the fear and dread these standard treatments hold for most people is based on the suffering they saw in the past. Almost thirty years ago I saw my own stoic father debilitated by intractable nausea after chemotherapy, weeping skin burns from chest radiation, and unyielding pain from shingles brought on by a weakened immune system. But he would not have had to suffer so now. There have been striking refinements in how a treatment is delivered, softened by near miraculous anti-nausea therapy, more controlled and targeted radiation technology, and effective means for sustained pain relief. The accelerating pace of change means that treatments given even five years ago may be less harsh today. As a result, cancer patients often don't need to drop out as they undergo cancer therapy. Treatment time is now a living time, too.

Surgery

When patients are told they have cancer, I think their first thought is *Take it out. Get rid of the alien that's of no use and wants to spread.* This is a logical thought and one that has guided cancer treatments over the ages. Surgery is the most obvious approach to tumors and has consistently proven to be curative over time—as long as the tumor is caught early and is fully removed. The natural history of an unchecked tumor fills the dusty old texts of medicine. Leave on a cancerous breast and it grows inflamed and ulcerated and takes over the body. Get the tumor out and there is a chance it is gone forever.

Etched into the papyrus of ancient Egypt are tales of the surgeon's knife in pursuit of cancer. Similar lore appears in the foundational medical teachings of ancient Greece and Rome. Eons before anesthesia, the agony of the scalpel was still seen as better for a patient than the cancer with which he was stricken. The first cancer surgery meant, for the most part, amputation—of a leg, an arm, or a breast. The intent was always to remove all the visible tentacles of the cancer spread, but success was often limited. Without the diagnostic tools of modern times, internal cancers before the last half century generally stayed hidden within the body, occasionally noted at autopsy. Most cancer victims just wasted away, without anyone knowing why.

John Hunter, the renowned eighteenth-century Scottish surgeon, wrote that surgery could cure cancer particularly if the tumor could be moved freely by the surgeon's hand, for that was a sign that it had not invaded. This was a rather astute observation, since invasion into nearby organs does mat (or, as it's often called, freeze) tissues together. Back then a cancer that invaded nearby was already too far gone for the surgeon's knife.

That changed. Radical surgery for cancer was in vogue in the middle of the last century. With better technology to support patients and blood transfusions to manage the major bleeding that often resulted, patients could survive the extensive surgical resections designed to root out every last bit of tumor. The results were often debilitating and disfiguring, leading surgeons such as George Crile Jr. to push for tissue-sparing surgery. Cancer researcher Bernard Fisher led a major NIH study that proved tissue-sparing lumpectomy was as effective as a deforming radical mastectomy in the treatment of early breast cancer. What made more limited surgery possible was the addition of the nonsurgical treatments, called adjuvant therapy, developed in the second half of the twentieth century. I must add that a huge part of the shift from radical surgery to lumpectomy came from women themselves, who wanted a say in their treatment and were willing to take the chance to opt for less as more.

Today, the cancer surgeon's work is most often combined with that of the radiotherapist, oncologist, or both, and combined with input from the patients themselves. Modern tools of the surgical trade now include miniature scopes and fiber-optic cameras that extend the surgeon's reach and view through the smallest of incisions. There are sonograms that guide biopsies precisely. We now have robotic three-dimensional guidance for deep and delicate surgery in areas from the brain to the prostate. In addition to the new reach and precision of these tools, recovery time and disability are shortened, sometimes dramatically.

There are still limits to what the knife can do. Even the slimmest blade works on the macroscopic level, while cancer lives on the micro level. It takes only a handful of seeds to start a garden, and no more missed cancer cells than that can spark recurrence. That's where radiation and chemotherapy come in. These mop-up treatments, able to neutralize much if not all of what's left behind, grew out of some of the greatest sleuthing in medical history. Ironically, for such lifesaving therapies, they were born of the great world wars.

Radiation Therapy

After Marie and Pierre Curie discovered radium in 1898, and Röntgen later turned the X-rays he discovered in 1895 to medical use, high doses of radiation were found to stop tumor growth cold. This led to high-dose radiation treatment for patients with end-stage cancer—so-called salvage therapy. Tumors shrank, but patients died with burns, infections, and bone marrow suppression. Refinements led to technology with the ability to deliver carefully dose-controlled radiation over a period of days to weeks, with less damage to normal tissue. A product of the wartime search for a substitute for radium, radioactive cobalt-60 appeared on the medical scene after World War II. The new radiation source was able to deliver ionizing gamma rays—the X-ray's higher-energy cousin—capable of penetrating tissues deeply with little or no injury to the skin surface.

Radiation targets localized tumor tissue and is presumed to work by its ionizing damage to DNA, a process that stops growth and triggers apoptosis. Now, through years of refinement, it has become a valuable first-line therapeutic choice for many localized cancers, including those of the prostate, head, neck, and brain. It's often used instead of surgery, and in combination with chemotherapy. Long and often painful experience has taught us about the damaging effects of radiation on surrounding normal tissue and its blood supply, leading to ever-better means for delivering it in narrower and more-focused beams.

This is the thinking behind brachytherapy (*brachy*- is Greek for "short"), in which numerous radioactive "seeds" or pellets are injected into a cancerous organ such as the prostate or uterus. This approach is used rather than radiating the area from afar with an external beam of radiation, a technique that cuts with a wider swath. The gamma knife used in brain surgery delivers a series of computer-directed cobalt beams that converge narrowly on the tumor. Intensity-modulated radiation therapy (IMRT) machines break radiation up into beamlets, delivered in three-dimensional arrays that match the shape of the tumor. The result is less radiation hitting the normal tissue around the tumor's edge with more intense doses delivered directly to the tumor. Even newer approaches combine the destructive power of radiation with the specificity of the immune system. In these new drugs, radioactive isotopes such as iodine are coupled to a highly specific antibody that latches on to a target molecule found only on the cancer cells, delivering radiation directly to the offending cells. One of these drugs, Bexxar (I-131 tositumomab), has shown promising results in one form of aggressive lymphoma.

Chemotherapy

Mustard gas was a deadly and feared chemical weapon first used in World War I. In 1919, after an accidental gas exposure during a military maneuver, doctors noticed that the exposed soldiers' white blood cell counts plunged and their lymphatic tissue shrank. The possibility that low doses of this dreaded agent might also decrease the dangerously elevated white blood cell counts of patients with leukemia eventually led researchers to design milder versions called nitrogen mustards, which could be injected into the veins. First used in patients in 1946, these chemotherapy agents radically changed cancer treatment and brought utter elation to a medical community virtually without options for the liquid tumors of the blood and for advanced, disseminated cancer. At Yale, Alfred Gilman and Frederick Philips injected these chemicals into patients with advanced lymphoma and watched in amazed satisfaction as their swollen lymph nodes shrank and their elevated white blood cell counts fell toward normal.

Though the benefit was temporary, this was a discovery moment that spawned numerous synthetic drugs fashioned to act in a similar way. Called alkylating agents, these drugs enter cells and form chemical bonds with strands of DNA, neatly tossing a monkey wrench into the gears of cell division. The injury sets the lifesaving process of cell suicide into motion. Today, these agents are a mainstay of chemotherapy; they include cyclophosphamide, melphalan, CCNU, chlorambucil, and Temodar (temozolomide), an important new drug that came of age while I was undergoing treatment.

Two years after nitrogen mustard first offered hope to lymphoma patients, Sidney Farber identified another drug, aminopterin, which worked in childhood leukemia. Like its chemical offspring methotrexate, which is still in use today, aminopterin stymied the growth of cancer cells by starving them of the vitamin folic acid, which is essential for making new DNA. Just imagine the miracle: children who had been dying, their blood vessels choked by millions of malignant white blood cells, suddenly went into remission. Farber's discovery was further proof that cancers could be controlled with medicine alone.

But it was with combinations of drugs, a concept introduced in the 1960s in the treatment of leukemia and lymphoma, that chemotherapy met with most success. Modeled after antibiotic therapy for bacterial infections, combination treatment uses several anticancer drugs at one time to prevent tumors from forming a resistance to any one drug. It's an approach that works well, but not always indefinitely. And that led to the next major advance in the treatment of these liquid cancers: bone marrow transplantation.

Bone Marrow Transplantation

Though the first line of attack for cancers of the blood and lymphatic system is still the multidrug chemotherapy cocktail, bone marrow transplantation is established therapy for relapsing disease. It has also been used experimentally in the treatment of some solid tumors with the aim of averting the spread of the cancer to other parts of the body. That's why my bone marrow stem cells were harvested and frozen when I first became ill. It was insurance; in the event that I did not respond to the initial chemotherapy, I would be prepared for at least one protocol that called for a different drug along with a bone marrow transplant.

Although the first successful bone marrow transplant for leukemia was carried out by E. Donnall Thomas in 1956—a feat for which he was awarded a Nobel Prize in 1990—the procedure was both arduous and risky, and for years it was performed at only a handful of major centers. Under the pioneering leadership of oncologist George Santos, the Johns Hopkins Hospital became one of those centers, and it was there in the early 1970s that I first encountered it.

As an assistant resident in medicine I was assigned to care for a tall, rugged teenage boy who had acute leukemia and was eligible for one of the newer bone marrow treatment protocols. All of us involved with him—the doctors, nurses, aides, technicians, and his large family—were buoyed with enthusiasm, convinced that his case had all the makings of a cure. He was quite a soldier; a stoic young man who never winced or complained as he spent months in a dreary isolation room, facing recurrent bouts of transplant rejection and a seemingly endless string of bone marrow biopsies. Not only was the transplant not "taking," but the new bone marrow, obtained from his sibling, began to attack his body with graft-versus-host disease. We watched helplessly as he succumbed to overwhelming pneumonia, a silent hero who made way for the patients of today, who face something very different.

One big advance came with the bioengineered drug Neupogen (filgrastim), which stimulates the new marrow to take root in a matter of days. This decreases not only the time in isolation but also the risk of infection. Neupogen, combined with better drugs to prevent and treat both transplant rejection and graft-versus-host disease, has made this procedure less risky and vastly less arduous for all involved. On the medical scorecard of advances in cancer treatment, bone marrow transplantation gets a gold star.

Treatment Is Personal

My own treatment was conventional, maybe even ancient. The FDA approved the newest drug in my PCV cocktail, CCNU, approximately thirty years ago; the oldest, vincristine, more than forty years ago; and procarbazine in 1969, with all three making their name in the conquest of Hodgkin's disease. The early successes with drugs, which brought with them serious side effects, made it clear that care of the cancer patient was no longer just about surgery; it called for the talents of a skilled team working together with expertise drawn from all corners of the hospital. From this emerged the dedicated cancer center providing an integrated approach to research and treatment.

Most elements of the modern medical campus carry welcoming names—heart institute, children's hospital, birthing center, wellness center, or center for sports medicine. By comparison, a cancer institute sounds dark and foreboding. I had trouble even getting the word *cancer* out. I called my illness a tumor, not a cancer; and the recently named Taussig Cancer Center simply the Taussig. Actually, Taussig is a rather beautiful and meaningful name for me. The center is named for a fallen soldier in the cancer war, honored after his death by a generous gift from his son, Brian Taussig, a young businessman in the community. I admired Brian and his wife's devotion to his father, and their generosity to others who needed cancer care. But truth be told, the name already had a warm and cozy spot in my heart.

Helen Taussig (no relationship to Brian) was the grand dame of cardiology, and the woman from Hopkins who discovered back in the 1950s how to turn blue babies pink again with a surgical procedure dubbed the Blaylock-Taussig operation. I came to know her in the later years of her life during the time I was at Johns Hopkins, and adored her utterly inspiring strength, fortitude, and equanimity. I guess she was my rock star. As a young physician in a medical world where women were scarce and their acceptance close to nil, she was assigned the grim job no one else wanted: caring for babies and children with congenital heart disease—the end-stage, hopeless cases, weak, blue, and dying of slow asphyxiation. But Dr. Taussig, studying the early developments in blood vessel surgery, figured out just how to help these most helpless of patients, and after many rejections finally convinced Dr. Alfred Blaylock, the head of surgery, to perform her rationally designed procedure. It worked, and it was a miracle, shooting around the world and opening up the whole field of congenital heart surgery. I remember watching stories of this triumph on our ten-inch black-and-white TV set as a little girl, marveling at the goodness of medical discovery. So on two counts Taussig is a hero's name, a word to inspire hope and courage. And hope and courage are palpable in the Taussig and many other places like it.

Whatever your tumor's name, there is a sameness in the people you see in the waiting rooms and elevators of cancer centers. We recognize each other at a glance, clutching our brown paper bags of medicines. A slower gait. A paleness that no artificial blush can hide. Hair thin or gone. The slim bodies, draped in newly oversized clothes. Our hosts, too, share many qualities. Cancer centers seem to attract teams of kind and empathetic staff, ready to help you with directions, draw your blood, patiently explain what to expect, lead support groups, and walk patients through their new routines. They also teach unexpected things, such as a dozen ways for the immunosuppressed to avoid infection, including stuffing purse or pockets with hand sanitizers; avoiding crowds, potted plants, flowers, and pepper; and shying away from children, ill family members, and household pets.

Eating is a big casualty of treatment. Sometimes the diet must be modified because of a particular drug, and your nurse advisor will tell you, for example, to avoid cheese or red wine, smoked fish or sauerkraut (as if a chemo patient has much appetite for such gourmet delights—low-grade nausea, joined by funny tastes and mouth ulcers, has a way of keeping noshing to a minimum). You quickly learn why bone marrow toxicity is the most serious side effect, as it sets you up for fatigue, infections, and bleeding. But the passel of side effects almost always resolves after treatment is completed, and I should point out that the newer gene-targeted drugs are not without their own side effects—ones that we are only beginning to understand. For example, Herceptin can trigger heart failure in as many as 4 percent of patients, and Avastin can bring on high blood pressure and blood clots.

On the positive side of this trek, you know the stuff is powerful, and in the great scheme of things, side effects are a steep but, under the circumstances, acceptable price for getting your life back. Taking on a cancer is serious business, and treatment often seems less bitter to the patient than to those who look on. I've found that most of us with cancer look beyond the treatment's difficulties, though of course we have little choice. Still, necessity brings a natural game face to this battle, a game face that has a focused edge, especially on those days when you are going to find out whether the gods have granted you a reprieve.

I felt that edge keenly the day I had my MRI scan after completing the first cycle of chemotherapy. It seemed as if a world of time had filled the eight weeks since my diagnosis. I was back at work, and life at home had settled into its old, delicious routines. I had successfully weathered one bout of bone marrow toxicity that troubled my bone marrow expert, Dr. Bolwell, more than it did me. Relieved and hopeful, I felt that I could do this treatment and still carry on with my life as if I were entirely well—I even kind of liked my new, smaller size. But scan time brought me back to cancer's reality.

My doctors warned me not to expect too much improvement after just one month of treatment, but this scan, and every repeat look inside my head, was still a kind of reckoning. I started the ordeal at the Taussig with a visit to Maureen Bell, my warmhearted oncology nurse, who drew some blood and flushed my port; then it was time to face the MRI. The drill is familiar to every patient who has ever had one: take off your watch and shoes and get positioned on the motorized bed that will slide you into a tunnel, where you must lie as still as a mummy for what in my case was a full hour of noisy scanning, for which I strongly recommend earplugs. There I lay, head rigid, arms fixed, eyes staring upward with nothing to see, encased in a sleek white sarcophagus. It's rather peaceful in there, but only if you force yourself to make it a time for quiet reverie, meditation, or even a little nap. Anyway, there wasn't much else I could do; there was no room in there for jumping out of my skin with anxiety.

I promptly came to life as the noise ceased and I was motored out of the narrow tunnel. There was my neurologist, Pat Sweeney, standing in the doorway right next to the computer console where the neuroradiologist, Dr. Paul Ruggieri, was studying the scan. Dr. Sweeney flashed a big smile and held both thumbs up. And behind him was my husband, looking on with his luscious grin. I had won a reprieve—the drugs were working sooner than expected, and the second cycle looked like no big deal.

But things don't always turn your way in medical treatment, and cancer, with its trial-and-error twists, offers far too many opportunities for something to go wrong. I hit a big speed bump early in my second cycle when I had a second and more serious run of bone marrow toxicity, which showed up clearly in my blood numbers. My platelets, key to blood clotting, fell to a few thousand from over 100,000 per microliter of blood, while the immunity-giving white cells plummeted to below 500 out of an expected 10,000. By then the oxygen-carrying red cells were deep in the anemic zone, but despite the ugly numbers I felt amazingly well. I popped the antibiotic Cipro to ward off infection, monitored my temperature, and gave in a bit more to the nagging fatigue that comes with anemia. If I felt weaker, I was buoyed by an even better MRI after cycle two, which showed that the tumor was seriously on the run.

My marrow, apparently, did not share my joy, and refused to bounce back as scheduled. Dr. Cohen comforted me with the medical folklore that such toxic reactions sometimes correlated with tumor wipeout. Even so, he joined the rest of my brain trust in agreement that my marrow could not tolerate a third bout of what's labeled grade IV marrow toxicity. Any more exposure to these drugs and I ran the risk of doing to my marrow what I hoped to do to my cancer, turning marrow-filled bones into barren cavities. The pit of my stomach quietly ached when in unison they said no more PCV, when I knew the plan had been for me to have five to six cycles.

These are the wrenching happenings that often occur along cancer's path. Yet in the medical textbooks and journal articles that I would regularly devour, they were little more than footnotes. When I found the sentence that mentioned the patients who had to discontinue treatment for toxicity, all I wanted to know was, "What then?" But for the authors of the study, they were mere dropouts. That did not help me with my dilemma one bit.

Here I was with a chemosensitive tumor that was melting away, and I could no longer take the miracle medicine that was doing the trick. My bone marrow was fighting with my brain, and the marrow stem cells I had so laboriously saved would be of no use, said my bone marrow maven, Dr. Bolwell. As he put it plainly, repeated damage can turn the marrow cavities into arid soil. You may have the seeds, but they will not grow if the marrow space is filled with scar tissue. With more of these treatments my bone marrow would be permanently destroyed, leaving me short on oxygen, short on blood-clotting ability, and devoid of an immune system. What a pickle, as my dad used to say.

But by sheer luck something else was happening. Temodar (temozolomide), the new drug developed by Schering-Plough, had just gained FDA approval for use in brain tumors that had failed to respond to other treatments; it would hit the pharmacy shelves in a matter of weeks. This was the first new drug to join the fight against brain tumors in decades, and it had a special knack for crossing the blood-brain barrier. And, crucially for me, Temodar delivered less bone marrow toxicity than PCV. I became one of its earliest users, and for the next year my scans steadily improved. Now, years later, this drug is recognized as a breakthrough in brain tumor treatment and is the first drug to be used routinely early in the treatment of glioblastoma multiforme, the most severe and common of the malignant brain tumors. For less common gliomas, like my oligo version, it's now standard care.

How easy it is to take new drugs for granted, especially when you don't need them. And it's entirely too easy to bash pharmaceutical companies for their profits, which sometimes may well be too steep, or for their drugs' side effects, which are never fully understood until a drug has been in use for many years. As all doctors know, drug discovery is the essential partner of medical practice, a major engine of progress and the ultimate translation of medical research into patient good. In my own field of the heart, blockbuster drugs to thin blood, lower blood pressure, and lower cholesterol transformed patient care. Now, as a patient myself, I found that a little-heralded drug, serving a mere handful of patients, made all the difference.

CHAPTER 11

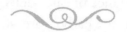

Treatment Scorecards

WHEN YOU'RE LIVING WITH cancer, a cure is the miracle you yearn for. There have been many incredible advances during the course of America's war on this disease; hundreds of thousands of dedicated scientists and clinicians have spent their careers getting us to where we are now. Despite these efforts, we are just beginning to tackle the really big problem: the way cancer kills.

The dramatic medical breakthroughs of the past forty years have moved overall cancer survival from about 50 percent to 65 percent, where it hovers today. This improvement looks even more modest when you consider that cancer survival rates are reported at the five-year mark. Five years without a recurrence is often taken as a cure. These are useful milestones for research purposes, but such benchmarks have less meaning to patients. To them, five years is a flash of time, and the way they live during it all-important. Whatever the

cancer type, to those facing cancer, a cure—or, almost as good, remission and control for their natural life span—is what counts for
them.

But before we declare the war on cancer a failure, we need to
take a closer look at the numbers. Going cancer by cancer, two dominant trends emerge, both of which can guide our future efforts. The
first is the primary importance of early detection. Lump together the
cancers that can be detected early—breast, prostate, colon, cervix,
thyroid, skin—and treatment scores have improved, often dramatically. Not perfect, but awfully good, as I will show later in this chapter. But look at the deep and hidden cancers that reveal themselves
in later stages—lung, pancreas, stomach, liver, and brain—and substantial improvement in treatment outcome still eludes us. These
hidden tumors show up in their own time, typically once they have
strangled or obstructed nearby tissues and organs, or grown to the
point where the tumor's fragile surface leaks blood or fluid into
places where it can be discovered. For these cancers, treatment may
prolong life, but the therapy is more intense, more debilitating, and
often less successful.

The second trend relates to the first: the greatest shortcoming of
cancer medicine today is its limited ability to tackle metastatic cancer. Disseminated cancer untouched by our current therapies accounts for most of the 500,000 deaths from the disease that occur
every year in the United States. Solving the problem of metastasis is
the single greatest challenge for cancer research.

To illustrate the cancer scorecard at its best and at its worst, let
me begin with one historical example: cervical cancer. With routine
use of Pap smears, cervical cancer deaths have plummeted. Yet this
cancer still devastates women today, particularly in many less-
developed parts of the world. Unchecked, cervical cancer freezes
the pelvic organs as it encircles and invades them in a great mass
of tumor. Treatment at that stage is pelvic exenteration, a radical
procedure in which the surgeon empties out the pelvis, including reproductive organs, bladder, and rectum, combined with radiation

treatments to quell the cancer's further spread. After all this, many of these women are only palliated—safe for the moment, but disfigured, debilitated, in pain, and facing a grim survival outlook that even today averages below 25 percent at five years.

Lesson from the Bedside

It was not so long ago when invasive cervical cancer was a common occurrence in this country, ravaging women in every nook of society. I remember that time well. During my years in medical school in the late 1960s, when I was a moonlighter in the blood bank of what was then called the Boston Hospital for Women, this disease seemed to be everywhere.

The Boston Hospital for Women, now part of Harvard's Brigham and Women's Hospital, was then a solitary place that specialized in non-obstetrical gynecology. Nestled in an out-of-the-way, quiet brick compound surrounded by arching old trees and expanses of lawn in a quaint residential area in Brookline, Massachusetts, it was a few miles' walk from the hustle and bustle of the medical school's towering all-purpose teaching hospitals. I worked in the small, one-room blood bank there as a round-the-clock weekend technician to draw patients' blood and type and cross-match their red cells with donated units for blood transfusions. When things were quiet I would go over to the adjacent nurses' residence and study in my on-call room, or chat with the nurses about some of the patients I'd encountered. It was a cozy place, and one that very much welcomed a female medical student, still a rarity in those days.

But radical surgery for advanced cervical cancer was not rare. Pelvic exenteration was a common procedure on Boston Women's operating room schedule, and that operation typically called for lots of blood. I got to know many women facing this surgery, since they had long hospital stays and many return visits. I was struck by how many were young, in their thirties and forties, with children at home, grieving in the long days and nights away from their families.

Most had been diagnosed only after experiencing the classic symptom of cervical cancer—post-coital bleeding, a sign that the tumor had become large enough to erode and inflame the cervix.

How vulnerable they were, shocked by what was happening to them, and so very much alone. They were emotionally isolated by their gynecologic cancers—such things were not spoken of much in polite company—and physically isolated in a hospital far away from the place that other cancer patients went for care. There was one woman in particular, in her late forties, who somehow became "my patient," something special for a young medical student anxious to move from the books to the bedside. She was elegant, reminding me by her looks and throaty voice of Lauren Bacall, and she wanted me to understand her illness. I'll call her Mrs. G.

One Saturday when I went in on a blood-drawing mission, Mrs. G. was disappointed that I had just missed the bride. Her daughter was to be married that afternoon, and she and her bridesmaids had come by in their wedding finery to see Mom beforehand. I wondered why she couldn't go herself, even in a wheelchair, at least for the ceremony. But with her throaty, confident voice and Boston accent, she said without flinching, "Dear, I cannot go. Not swimming in this sea of shit." She jarred me into reality; I saw her only as a beautiful, proper, and heroic woman taking on a tough problem, not as a gaunt, anemic patient struggling in pain, with a leaking and infected colostomy tube. I felt so awkward and inadequate, very much the kid, not the doctor, bungling into a place I didn't want her to have to go. I never saw her again; this was her dying time. She had just kissed her daughter good-bye. She left me, someone who barely knew her, with an embrace, too: a burning image of a lonely patient sequestered in a "woman's hospital" and dying of a disease she never needed to have. Mrs. G. was born too early.

Since that time her medical story has become the exception rather than the rule. Because Pap smears are now embedded in women's routine health care, most cervical cancer is detected long before any symptoms appear. When the disease is picked up early, before it has started to spread, a minor outpatient surgical procedure can core out the ring of bad cells at the junction of the cervix and uterus, curing the disease and leaving the womb and fertility intact. Early invasive cancer can be cured with a hysterectomy—a serious procedure and one that robs a childbearing-age woman of her fertility, but vastly preferable to exenteration.

This triumph of early detection has now been matched by another: cervical cancer has become one of the few cancers whose cause is known. As noted earlier, certain strains of the sexually transmitted HPV virus, which can silently incubate in the cervix for years, attack the DNA of infected cervical cells and set them on cancer's path. And from that insight into the mechanism of the disease has come the two preventive vaccines, Cervarix and Gardasil, to immunize women against these known cancer-producing strains. In time HPV vaccination should send cervical cancer the way of smallpox—here and around the world.

For now, however, we are still faced with the harsh reality of metastatic cancer. Were Mrs. G. afflicted with her advanced disease even today, we would have little more to offer her now than we did back then. The options for treating widespread disease such as hers have not advanced much beyond better means for pain relief. In the United States alone, and despite the wide availability of Pap smears, close to 4,000 women a year are still dying her death.

As I go on to review the most common cancers we face today, you will see these same themes repeated again and again. One caveat here: I will be using survival rates at five years only because in the common language of oncologists and epidemiologists, used to compare outcomes based on anatomic site, grade, and stage, five years without recurrence is often taken as a cure. These measures provide a general index of tumor behavior and effectiveness of current treatment. But I caution, as I do throughout this book, that these averages have wide spreads and can fail miserably as a crystal ball for any one person.

Lung Cancer

Lung cancer leads as the single most common cancer killer of men and women worldwide. It lacks an established means of early detection, and that, combined with what is often a fast-growing aggressive tumor, explains why 95 percent of the men and women who receive that diagnosis are slated to die of the disease. In the United States alone it claims 163,000 lives per year, despite the 15 percent decline in lung cancer deaths over the past decade, attributed mainly to a decline in smoking among men. Women lag, with only a recent leveling off of what has been a steady increase in lung cancer deaths since the late 1960s. To the surprise of many, it is the lung, not the breast, that accounts for most cancer deaths in women. Another surprise is that 30 percent of those with lung cancer have never smoked, and more women than men fall into this group.

Still, it's lifelong smokers, such as the former ABC news anchor Peter Jennings, who make up the bulk of lung cancer patients. This vigorous, otherwise healthy man developed hoarseness, which seemed like nothing at first. But when triggered by lung cancer, a rasp in the voice signals advanced disease. He is like many millions of others, including my own father, in whom this tumor took off seemingly out of the blue, quickly ravaging his entire body.

As a young cardiologist at Hopkins, I picked up Dad's illness immediately when I heard his suddenly raspy voice on the telephone; he told me of just then waking up with a swollen face, a classic sign of tumor blocking the veins from the head emptying into the heart. My dad, who came of age when cigarettes were cool and cartons were sent as holiday gifts, stopped smoking when I was in medical school. He said it was a direct result of my bringing home a pathology textbook to show him the cancer's ugly pictures. Though he went cold turkey at age fifty, by then he had racked up more than seventy pack-years (two packs per day since age fourteen). That hefty cumulative dose of carcinogens took his life eighteen months after he fell ill at the age of sixty-eight. And since we lost him more than two decades ago, the cure rate of the disease has not gotten much better.

The vast majority of patients with lung cancer have their disease picked up only when it is already advanced. They face surgery, chemotherapy, and radiation and still have a poor record of survival—15 percent at five years overall. For those fortunate enough to have their disease detected when it is localized to the lung—and that's almost always because of an incidental finding while doing a chest X-ray or scan for something else—survival averages better than 50 percent. But if the cancer has spread extensively by the time it comes to medical attention because of a raspy voice, unexplained cough, or blood in the sputum, survival plummets to under 5 percent.

What frustrates doctors is that the gold standard for diagnosis of lung disease, the chest X-ray, misses 85 percent of stage I cancers, the earliest, smallest, most localized tumors that have no symptoms and are the most easily treatable and curable. There is now a chance to change this—to turn lung cancer from a "have-not" to a "have"— if the medical community gets on board with a new program just recently validated for easy and efficient lung cancer screening. The final work was reported in late 2006, and involved cancer centers from around the world working together as part of the International Early Lung Cancer Action Program (I-ELCAP), centered at Cornell. Despite some astounding findings, the application of its screening approach to the biggest cancer killer on the planet is being caught up in a pulmonary version of the mammogram wars.

The long-awaited international study screened more than 30,000 symptom-free people at high risk for lung cancer, mostly because they were smokers. Using rapid CT scans that deliver low-dose radiation comparable to that of a mammogram, hidden cancers were found mostly in the earliest stages of growth. Overall estimated ten-year (not five-year) survival rate for all CT-scanned patients was 80 percent in I-ELCAP. For those in stage I who were treated with prompt surgery, it was over 90 percent.

Just imagine what this could mean: 130,000 people a year in the United States alone could be saved, according to Dr. Claudia Henschke, the professor of radiology at Cornell's Weill Medical College, who led the thirteen-year study. In perspective, that's more than the number of people lost to breast, prostate, and colon cancer *combined* every year. And it opens the door to consider lumpectomy rather than lobectomy for the smallest of tumors, reaping better lung function for cancer survivors—provided that minimal surgery does not diminish cure rate.

There's been a barrage of criticism that widespread population screening will lead to unneeded lung biopsies and operations on tumors that are not really dangerous—the very same arguments that are still used ad nauseam against mammograms and PSA screening. But in the I-ELCAP protocol, only those patients with scans that have a high certainty of being cancer (based on size, shape, and growth) are biopsied. What doctors would not biopsy a small mass that looks like a cancer and is growing before his or her eyes, even if it is only millimeter by millimeter? As a result, in I-ELCAP, better than 90 percent of the biopsies performed found cancer. If patients and doctors can be assured of the same quality of technology and expertise, moving forward now with such screening is just common sense.

The Lung Cancer Alliance is enthusiastic about what it sees as a dramatic breakthrough for patients and is encouraging high-risk patients to talk to their doctors. But these health champions are all too often unheard. Over the years members of the Alliance have told me about the difficulty of getting their concerns across to the public as well as to policy makers. Part of the reason, they fear, is that too many people cling to the idea that if you have lung cancer you've brought it on yourself by smoking cigarettes. It's somehow not politically correct to rally for this disease. Recently, the Alliance has been running ads to show the public that even nonsmokers just like themselves get this disease, too. Indeed, we all know of Christopher Reeve's wife, Dana, who died in 2006 at age forty-four of lung cancer. She never smoked. Neither did a respected colleague of mine, the cancer researcher, Nobel Prize winner, and longtime anti-smoking activist from the University of Wisconsin, Howard Temin, who died at the age of fifty-nine from lung cancer.

Stigmas are never good. But more important, here they obscure the reality that cancer is a disease of the human condition that at this point in time takes its greatest toll in the form of lung cancer. In the past it was cervical cancer in women. In that sense, the Lung Cancer Alliance leads a common cause for reducing deaths from cancer in our population, and finding ways to counter advanced disease.

Breast Cancer

I suspect no woman is entirely free from the fear that breast cancer will be hers one day. Virtually all of us have a family member, friend, or loved one who has faced this disease. It's the most common cancer in women, with 275,000 new cases a year in the United States, including 62,000 new cases of in-situ or pre-invasive disease. Some 41,000 women and 460 men die of advanced disease yearly.

The widespread use of mammograms, however much they have been criticized, has vastly improved breast cancer's scorecard. Even when breast cancer is invasive within the breast, overall survival to five years now approaches 100 percent; it is about 80 percent when the cancer has spread to lymph nodes. We have to credit women's activism for our heightened awareness of the disease, for the fact that most women follow the current early screening guidelines, and also for their public support of major research investments. This includes the Women's Health Initiative, which among other things is now being credited for a recent and dramatic one-year drop of 7 percent in new diagnoses of breast cancer. Many scientists are attributing the decline to reduced use of hormonal therapy among menopausal women. This came in the wake of widely published research showing that women who took combination HRT had a significant increase in the disease after as little as five years.

Breast cancer research has long laid the tracks for translating basic biological insights into treatment, with its early recognition of the role of estrogen in stimulating receptor-positive breast cancer cells to grow and for developing strategies to block its effect. Decades ago that was done by removing a pre-menopausal woman's ovaries; now it is done ever so much more precisely with designer drugs such as tamoxifen and more recently the aromatase inhibitors.

The secrets of breast cancer really started to open up when scientists decoded the genes *BRCA1* and *BRCA2*, to explain why the cancer runs in 5–10 percent of families. On the treatment side, the discovery of the gene *HER2/neu* provided a way to predict an especially aggressive form of breast cancer. It also became the template for targeted drugs such as Herceptin and more recently Tykerb (lapatinib), which cut down on recurrence and metastases in those women who have the gene.

With these therapeutic breakthroughs, breast cancer patients are seeing some improvement in survival for advanced disease, which is now about 25 percent. Even so, this number reminds us again that metastatic disease calls for researchers to go back to the biological drawing board. On this score, the breast cancer field may again be leading the way with some pioneering work in the area of cancer-bearing stem cells. As a reminder, these are not the controversial embryonic stem cells perpetuated in the laboratory, but adult stem cells that are naturally occurring in all of us to help our bodies repair and restore injured or tired tissue.

Cancerous stem cells have been clearly identified in breast cancer, and recent studies suggest they are the cells that are behind the growth, spread, and recurrence of this disease. Once we get more information on the altered genome of these hidden cells, we could develop an entirely new double-barreled treatment strategy: existing therapies would be used to wipe out the tumor mass and a new targeted therapy would knock out the small number of hidden cancer stem cells—the tumors' seeds that cause spread and recurrence. This two-front attack would also be relevant to other malignancies that have been shown to harbor cancer-initiating stem cells, including those of the prostate, brain, head and neck, and maybe ovary and pancreas, as well as cancers of the blood.

Prostate Cancer

If you are a boomer or beyond, you can't go anywhere without hearing about yet another man just diagnosed with prostate cancer. This is the most frequently detected cancer in men, with some 235,000 men diagnosed with this disease annually. But the good news is that this cancer boasts one of the best scores for both control and cure. And for that, early detection and treatment once again get the credit.

No doubt there are biological factors that have contributed to this success as well. Topping the list is that in most men the tumor grows slowly. And as we now are able to detect this cancer in its earliest stages, even in an in-situ form, there is often a dilemma as to timing for treatment. Do you move quickly to prostatectomy, which can have side effects on bladder control and sexual function, or just wait? We are learning about tumor gene profiles that make some prostate cancers more aggressive in some young men, but they are not yet ready to be a certain guide for therapy. Watchful waiting, the practice of monitoring men who have known prostate cancer, is an acceptable approach in older men.

Recent studies have shown that watchful waiting is more bold than right for younger men, in particular. In a recent ten-year analysis, prostate cancer patients under the age of sixty-five lived significantly longer with a prostatectomy and suffered substantially less local progression and distant spread of their cancers compared to those who chose watchful waiting. Those who opted to let the tumor take its course experienced more medical problems and a lesser quality of life, including trouble urinating and pain from tumor spread, particularly to the bones.

Even those without evident progression of the disease wrestled with the anxiety of knowing that the tumor could be silently ticking away. The differences were not as great among men whose tumors were discovered when they were over sixty-five, but the results of this study and others still favor prostate removal. What should be most comforting is that the five-year survival rate is reported at 100 percent for both localized and regional prostate cancer. When metastatic disease occurs, five-year survival is in the range of 35 percent—again, the weak spot in our cancer scorecard.

Prostate and breast cancer have many similarities. Both are stimulated by sex hormones, both produce slower-growing tumors in the elderly, and many of the genes that are linked to breast cancer, such as *BRCA1* and *BRCA2*, also increase the risk of prostate cancer in men. Hormonal therapy that blocks testosterone plays a big role in the treatment of prostate cancer, much as anti-estrogen treatment does for breast cancer. Thus far, however, other forms of chemotherapy have not, though this may be changing as newer approaches to chemotherapy, and immunotherapy using vaccines, are showing promise for more advanced disease.

Men have also followed on the heels of women in expecting treatment choices. Options include surgery, radiation of the gland, or, as mentioned, watchful waiting with hormonal treatment. Nerve-sparing surgery and newer developments with robot-guided prostate removal have diminished the side effects of prostatectomy. Because of continued concern about nerve injury related to both prostate removal and radiation, new procedures that destroy the cancerous tissue with lasers or freezing have been developed, although it's still too early to be sure how they stack up in terms of cure.

Colon Cancer

Some of cancer's biggest research scores are drawn from work on the many forms of colon cancer that run in families. Scientists have learned about inherited as well as accumulating genetic mistakes that lead to the cancer's development and progression. At the same time—and providing the needed cancer tissue to do this research—

was the engineering feat that made colon cancer a model of cure through early detection. The feat, of course, is the fiber-optic colonoscope, which enables doctors to visually scan the entire inside lining of the colon and rectum through a flexible tube in a matter of minutes, exposing the tiniest of polyps—the red flag of cancer in waiting. Only through the many clinical studies of polyps removed from patients at all stages of the disease did doctors learn that these little pre-cancerous protrusions from the inner colon wall are the common denominator of this disease. Get them small and get them out and the patient is cured—a major breakthrough for the third most common cancer in the United States.

If a small polyp contains a nest of cancerous cells that have not yet invaded into the wall beneath the bowel lining, removal at colonoscopy along with frequent colon examinations thereafter is all that's necessary to keep patients cancer free. Large polyps are most likely to bear invasive cancer and sometimes are big enough to require surgery with a partial colectomy. Even then, survival is about 90 percent. But if allowed to remain, polyps will grow slowly and silently until they signal their presence with blood in the stool, or more dramatically with an obstructed or perforated bowel. Then survival falls to about 70 percent if the cancer is still localized, but to less than 10 percent if it has spread to the liver and beyond.

Despite our current ability to actually prevent colon cancer from developing, there are still 149,000 cases of colorectal cancer a year in the United States. The disease has an overall five-year survival of 64 percent and causes 55,000 deaths annually. These scores are by no means what they could or should be. Does this mean this is one instance where preventive screening doesn't work? Unequivocally no. Instead, as the American Cancer Society reports, less than 40 percent of cancers are picked up early, because people avoid colon cancer screening.

When this cancer hits with invasive disease, patients face major therapy with surgery, radiation, and/or chemotherapy. What people who forgo their regular screening need to know is that treatment for a cancer that has spread through the bowel wall is a heck of a lot more arduous than a colonoscopy.

Beyond the Big Four

The American Cancer Society estimates that 1.4 million Americans face a diagnosis of invasive cancer each year. About 565,000 men and women will die—that is, 1,500 people a day. The "big four"—cancers of the lung, breast, prostate, and colon—make up about half of all these cancers and account for half of all cancer deaths. But beyond these four are legions more, each with its own natural history, biology, genomics, and pattern of response to therapy. Most of the attention, awareness, and research dollars go to the cancers that affect the most people; that makes sense. But this leaves many cancers—and cancer patients—as veritable orphans in the world of treatment.

About a year ago I read a small story in the back pages of the newspaper about a handful of patients with brain cancer who assembled to walk together at the very same time a massive race for the cure of breast cancer was under way. They wanted people to be aware of their cancer, too. I mention them not because I shared their illness, though that may have been the jolt that kept them in my mind, but more to point out that cancer has a very broad base made up of a wide range of tumors that people rarely hear about or think about—unless that tumor becomes their own.

With this in mind, I've listed several other cancers to illustrate the diversity of the disease called cancer; each tumor has its own unique twist. This recounting, which is by no means encyclopedic, makes it obvious how easy it is for a patient, doctor, or researcher to be isolated in a silo of their own disease. Yet it also shows common traits across many cancers, pointing to general principles that, if anything, should bind those of us with cancer together, scientifically as well as emotionally.

Pancreatic and Other Gastrointestinal Cancers

As we celebrate the advances in colon cancer, we should not forget that treatments of most cancers of the gastrointestinal system do not match its success. At the risk of repetition, it is mostly because we don't have the technology to catch them early. These are "have-not" tumors that lack early screening technology. Such is the case for stomach cancer, esophageal cancer, and cancer of the pancreas. The last of these has an overall five-year survival rate of less than 5 percent, unchanged in thirty years.

Pancreatic cancer kills over 30,000 Americans each year and ranks number five among deaths from cancer in this country. Even when found as a small localized tumor, current treatments are often disappointing. This has led some oncologists to theorize that early detection might not make much difference, because unusual tumor biology makes pancreatic cancer resistant to conventional cancer treatment. This biology might relate to stem cells. Scientists have now identified a distinctive molecular signaling pathway in human pancreatic cancer cells studied in the laboratory. Whimsically named Hedgehog, it normally plays a role in stem cell maintenance in early embryonic development of the pancreas, brain, lung, and prostate, and then shuts off, but it is again activated in some cancers later developing in these organs. Since more than 70 percent of pancreatic cancers show abnormalities of Hedgehog signaling, novel drugs are being fashioned to shut Hedgehog down, thus interrupting the cancerous cells' growth. One compound, cyclopamine, a natural plant steroid, does this in the lab, and has set off a search for less toxic forms of the agent.

This may sound like too much promise and not enough action for a deadly malignancy, but it's the very kind of work that is critical to solving the riddles of the "neglected" cancers. Such lines of discovery will surely impact on other types of cancer, and as the cycle time from discovery to application has shortened, key discoveries rarely languish in the lab for long.

Another gastrointestinal tumor, liver cancer, has a notoriously poor outcome, and the cancer is on the rise in the United States and worldwide. For a breakthrough, we must look to those working in infectious disease. It is the silent epidemic of hepatitis C that drives liver cancer. There is now a test to screen the virus out of the blood supply, which for years had been a source of infection of blood transfusion recipients. Progress is also being made on a vaccine to prevent the disease in the first place, much like the new hepatitis B vaccine already in use.

Ovarian Cancer

A swollen waistline, not a rare occurrence in women as they get older, is often the first sign that ovarian cancer's aggressive clones have already spread and are weeping a plasma-like fluid into the abdomen. This is still too often the way that the 20,000 new cases of ovarian cancer are detected each year, mostly in women over fifty. And because of that 15,000 women die each year. Routine screening rarely picks up ovarian cancer early; the ovaries are small and hidden deep in the pelvis, and they often shed their cancerous cells before a mass is obvious on physical exam or even by ultrasound.

Nevertheless, pelvic ultrasound, along with the blood tumor marker CA-125, is used routinely in women with a family history of the disease or who carry genes known to increase their risk. While they are not seen as reliable or efficient screening tests for the general population, they are the best we have.

The FDA and the National Cancer Institute have reported on blood protein patterns that can pick up early disease with great precision in over 95 percent of women who have it. They have not been released for use, however, for high-risk women, despite the fact that patients in whom the tumor is discovered early have a survival rate of 95 percent. (For the rest, it's between 30 and 70 percent, depending on how far the tumor has spread.) The arguments that keep early screening technology in the laboratory are variants of ones that are slowing down the use of low-dose CT for lung cancer, namely concerns that the test could lead to false positive results and unnecessary testing.

With so poor a scorecard for early detection, it's no surprise that prophylactic removal of the ovaries has become an acceptable personal option for high-risk women who have had their children—or for post-menopausal women, who not infrequently opt for a hysterectomy with this in mind.

Kidney and Bladder Cancer

The kidneys are nestled deep behind the organs of the gastrointestinal tract and can become enlarged, cystic, or even cancerous without a hint of a problem. Rather common signs, such as back pain or microscopic evidence of blood in the urine, lead to the cancer's discovery, but again, there is no early screening technology. We know that when the disease is diagnosed early, removing the cancerous kidney can be an easy cure. Even with local spread, survival is about 60 percent. But once the cancer has disseminated to the brain, survival falls to 15 percent or less.

This tumor, along with malignant melanoma, has some unique properties related to the immune system. Both have become a kind of bellwether for advances in immunotherapy. These tumors benefit from administration of the body's natural immune defense proteins interleukin-2 and interferon-alpha. Kidney cancer and also melanoma are tumors in which immunotherapy using vaccines still looks promising, inducing in some patients remarkable regression of tumors. But this is unpredictable and happens only in a handful of those treated. Until researchers can figure out more precise predictors of treatment outcome, the therapy will be stalled, but the enthusiasm for immunotherapy, which makes such intuitive sense, will not. Advanced cancer also benefits from new targeted drugs: a new agent, Sutent (sunitinib), a tyrosine kinase inhibitor, shrinks otherwise resistant metastatic renal cell tumors, and offers promise for earlier-stage disease.

Another genitourinary malignancy that sneaks up on patients is bladder cancer. It grows slowly both wide and deep, sometimes invading the muscle of the bladder wall before it is noticed because of pain or bloody urine. More than 61,000 people are diagnosed with this tumor annually, most of them in their later years. It strikes men three times more often than women, and smokers twice as often as nonsmokers. Treatment involves surgery and chemotherapy; superficial tumors can sometimes be treated locally through a cystoscope, a fiber-optic tube threaded into the bladder. With this, the overall five-year survival rate is 82 percent. When the cancer has spread to a distant organ, it falls to 6 percent. As I discussed in Chapter 8, a urine test for this cancer has won FDA approval, having been shown to be both lifesaving and cost-effective for high-risk symptom-free people. However, it has not yet become a routine part of regular cancer screening.

Cancers of the Blood and Lymphatic System

Leukemia and lymphoma are classified as "liquid cancers," because they involve cells that normally float in the fluids of the blood vessels and lymph ducts. In fact, these cancers have their origin in more hidden solid spaces: the marrow of the bones or the network of lymph nodes, where the cancerous stem cells grow.

Leukemia is a white blood cell cancer that is diagnosed in 35,000 people each year. Its outcome varies based upon which of several white blood cell types has become cancerous. Though we often hear about childhood leukemia, the disease is ten times more common in adults. Leukemia was among the first cancers to show the worth of chemotherapy, and progress continues with newer drugs and easier and safer bone marrow transplantation. One of the greatest successes has come with acute lymphocytic leukemia, which in the 1970s had five-year survival rates of 38 percent; today it's 65 percent, and for children survival rates are over 85 percent. Another reason for optimism is targeted drugs such as Gleevec, and the recently approved Sprycel (dasatinib), which bring remarkable remissions to patients with chronic myelogenous leukemia and other forms of Philadelphia chromosome-positive leukemia.

Hodgkin's lymphoma, which affects nearly 8,000 people annually, most in their teens and twenties, can be cured even if the cancer has spread into several lymph node regions. This is in contrast to non-Hodgkin's lymphoma, which is eight times more common, arises in an older population, and has a lower cure rate. Since the 1970s the incidence of this disease has doubled in the U.S. population, primarily among women. Non-Hodgkin's lymphoma took Jacqueline Kennedy Onassis's life at a relatively young age in 1994.

Since then, we have learned of the mixed array of risk factors for this disease, including compromised immune function, infection with a human T-cell leukemia/lymphoma virus, *H. pylori* infection of the stomach (the same bacterium that causes ulcers) for gastric lymphoma, and even a family history of lymphoma. Great progress has been made in using genetic and molecular technology to uncover unique gene signatures that are both predictive of disease progression and helpful in directing therapy. A specific gene pattern, for example, is now used routinely to assess outcome and treatment for patients with non-Hodgkin's B-cell lymphoma.

Multiple myeloma, a cancer of the antibody-producing white blood cells called plasma cells, is also increasing in frequency, particularly in the baby-boom generation. Showing up in 17,000 patients each year, it almost exclusively affects those over the age of fifty, steadily increasing its incidence with each subsequent decade of life. Smoldering for years, myeloma moves into an aggressive later stage where it chokes the bone marrow and clogs the kidney with heavy protein products. Unlike other liquid cancers, it can also infiltrate bone with tumors called plasmacytomas. Treatment combines chemotherapy with steroids, and this tumor has been one of the first to show the benefits of blocking tumor blood supply to stop its growth. The anti-angiogenesis agent thalidomide is now routine therapy for multiple myeloma. The newer agent Velcade (bortezomib), which targets the cancer cell's suicide program, has led to remarkable remissions. But myeloma is a classic case of cancerous cells skilled at quickly reengineering themselves to resist drug therapy; the goal is to find ways to stretch out the drug-induced remissions.

Brain Cancer

I am but one of the 360,000 people in the United States who live with the diagnosis of a tumor of the central nervous system (CNS). And every year 18,820 people will join our ranks because they have been found to have a malignant tumor of the brain. Overall five-year survival of those with brain and CNS tumors is 30 percent. But the survival rate is closer to 3 percent if the tumor is a glioblastoma multiforme (GBM), the most common primary brain tumor in adults. For the longest time this tumor has been cast as hopeless, but recently—very recently—things have begun to change. I've mentioned the mainstream bias against chemotherapy for brain tumors, but chemo's value for GBM is looking up in response to several gene-driven surprises, not unlike the gene discoveries that led to my own remission almost a decade ago.

GBM, which is also called a grade IV astrocytoma, is famous for its roaming cells, typical of stem cells, which pop up at the original site or in other parts of the brain within a matter of months. Standard therapy has been surgery and radiation; chemotherapy has been used as salvage treatment, a last-ditch effort after the tumor has recurred. But now the drug Temodar, which was so helpful to me, prolongs survival in patients with GBM when it's combined with standard radiotherapy. It's as if the drug makes the tumor more sensitive to destruction by radiation. Furthermore, researchers are just now identifying subtypes of GBM tumors that influence choice of therapy. For example, those with an abnormality in a gene called *MGMT*, which ordinarily repairs DNA, seem to benefit most from the drug-radiation combination. Another variant of this tumor lacks a tumor suppressor gene, *PTEN*, and overexpresses a form of the EGFR protein. In this subgroup, the addition of the new EGFR inhibitors such as Tarceva (erlotinib) has produced dramatic tumor shrinkages. And yet another abnormal gene pattern involving the vitamin A receptor has led oncologists to add the acne drug Accutane in that subset of patients. Velcade (bortezomib) and the anti-angiogenic drug Avastin (bevacizumab) also show promise.

Gene-driven chemotherapy has brought a renewed sense of energy to the once-dispirited field. This will only be accelerated as the NCI and National Human Genome Research Institute proceed with the Cancer Genome Atlas project, which has designated GBM as one of the three cancers whose entire genetic blueprint will be mapped in the first ongoing phase of this effort. Mapping GBM's genome, combined with the recognition of cancerous stem cells as the seeds of brain tumor development and recurrence, has put brain cancer research at the vanguard of the new cancer biology.

Children's Cancers

As cruel as it seems, cancer hits children, too. In the United States, after accidents, cancer is the leading cause of death among those between five and fifteen years of age. While their elders are afflicted mostly by carcinomas, the 9,000 new cases of childhood cancer that occur each year are, in order of frequency, leukemia, tumors of the brain and nervous system, and sarcomas that develop in places such as bone or muscle. None of these cancers can be blamed on the little ones' behavior or that of their parents, or on environmental exposures other than an unusual exposure to ionizing radiation. Rather, these cancers are simply inexplicable, thought to arise because of some random accident in early development.

As harsh as cancer in a child may be, the good news is that the cancer war has shown some of its most striking successes in children. Childhood leukemia and many a brain tumor can be cured. The overall five-year survival rate for childhood cancer is now 75 percent. Today, pediatric oncologists are focusing on achieving cures without the long-term side effects of treatment. For example, the use of whole-brain radiation, which impairs intellectual development, has largely been abandoned in cases of childhood leukemia— without substantially diminishing the favorable outcome.

Most children with childhood cancers are treated within the framework of NIH-sponsored clinical trials, and scientists will quickly tell you that this is why the field has been so successful. See Chapter 13 for more information on accessing clinical trials.

Metastatic Cancer

A scan of the cancer scorecard shows clearly that modern medicine is far less successful once the disease has spread to distant organs. This has led to a medical and research bias that paints metastatic cancer as a hopeless, end-stage disease rather than a universal stage of cancer progression that bears its own unique characteristics, which if understood and targeted would be treatable. This is not a pipe dream. In fact, in the early years of the cancer war, doctors were buoyed with optimism that advanced cancer would be cured, and that was based on some early and extraordinary successes.

In the early days of chemotherapy, when doctors were heady with the notion that medicine could push leukemia into complete remission, it was imagined that the same would be possible for disseminated solid tumors. One tumor fueled that expectation. It was an aggressive cancer that spread from the uterus to riddle the lungs, liver, and brain with metastatic tumors, snuffing out women's lives sometimes in a matter of months. In one of NIH's finest—and most unexpected—discoveries, this cancer in its disseminated state was found to melt away when young medical researcher Min Chiu Li, working with oncologist Roy Hertz in the mid-1950s, administered a chemotherapy that had a great track record helping children with leukemia but no track record with solid tumors. The response was so fast and so dramatic that some observers thought it was one of those rare cases of spontaneous remission. Yet, again and again, in other women stricken with the same cancer, the leukemia drug made the tumor disappear, returning its victims to perfect health as if the tumor had never been there. I vividly remember hearing of these remarkable cures when I was in medical school, and how stirred I was by the sense that any advanced cancer might be cured if only we found the right drug.

One would think that decades later, and thirty-five years into the official declaration of the war on cancer, that would now be the case. In retrospect this particular cancer had some unusual biological feature that made it vulnerable: it grew out of a pregnancy gone wrong, derived from the germ cells. Called choriocarcinoma, it occurs when the primitive stem cell tissue of the early embryo turns into a cancerous mass of placenta inside the womb, instead of forming a fetus. Most people have never heard of this once deadly tumor; today it affects 3,000 women a year, most of whom are cured and can go on to have normal pregnancies.

But most people have heard of a tumor that develops out of germ cells in men, too: testicular cancer, which affects 8,000 men annually, but each year takes fewer than 400 lives. With treatment, even men with the most advanced metastatic disease riddling the belly, lungs, and brain undergo near-miraculous cures. From that perspective, Lance Armstrong, one of the best-known men who had this disease, is far more than the usual cancer survivor. He is living proof that metastatic cancer, too, can be cured, leaving the patient unscathed, if only we find the right treatment.

Today's failures with most other forms of metastatic cancer have led to the unfortunate belief that this is invariably end-stage disease. But molecular studies are teaching us that cancers at different stages have distinct biological features. Metastatic disease takes on properties of mobility and distant growth that in themselves stand out as targets. This calls for an integrated research effort that cuts across the tumor "silos" that keep doctors and researchers focused on one cancer from working or communicating with those focused on another. It also calls for more research dollars and other resources devoted to understanding and treating metastatic disease. Why is our investment relatively skimpy when in fact it is this stage of disease that is responsible for most of cancer's pain, suffering, and loss of life? This must change. And it will if two of today's hottest areas of medical research get enough attention: the matrix that surrounds and supports cancer spread, and the adult stem cells that may seed its destruction.

The march and invasion of metastatic cancer cells depends on well-developed matrix-invasion powers, including a targeted command of the host's immune system, the ability to create a new blood supply, and the skill to drill holes in structures as tough as bone. This is the promise of anti-angiogenic agents, anti-inflammatory treatments, and immunotherapy. Even matrix-strengthening agents bring benefit, such as the intravenously administered forms of the bone-building bisphosphonates. The oral form of these drugs, such as Fosamax (alendronate) and Didronel (etidronate), are well known to women with osteoporosis because they block bone breakdown, which is precisely what occurs when metastatic cancer cells punch holes in the skeleton to set up their own shop. What a pleasant surprise when doctors discovered that this approach, which is used in advanced breast and prostate cancer as well as in multiple myeloma, makes bones more resistant to cancer invasion and cuts down on bone pain.

As for cancer stem cells, we have only begun to explore the nature of these cancerous seeds. Decoding the genome of cancer stem cells will point toward therapies that might ward off metastatic disease long before the first cell sets up residence in a distant site. The science is ripe, the genomics revolution is here, and the number of people who will be lost due to metastatic cancer is destined to rise as our population ages. But an assault on metastatic cancer will take a collaborative mind-set and an intense commitment of talent and resources.

Looking Ahead: A Public Scorecard

A cancer scorecard ultimately comes with only one name on it. We all want our own cancer cured, but that success is very much dependent on advances with other forms of cancer as well. That's why it is ultimately a war on cancer that will be won, not a fragmented war on two hundred cancers waged independently. If you are under eighty-five, cancer, not heart disease, will most likely be your biggest health issue. With the speed of discovery enabled by modern technology, almost everyone should expect to see developments in the next few years that will benefit them personally.

Practically speaking, the payoffs will come in two dimensions. The "have-not" cancers must become "haves." That is, all tumors deserve to be detected early, and gene-based molecular markers float-ing in the blood or body fluids and safe, high-resolution imaging technology will get us there. At the same time, we cannot abandon the sick. We can make cancer no more than a chronic disease if we master the secrets of advanced, resistant, and metastatic disease, whatever its first cell of origin. As this brief recounting has made clear, this is where the scorecard is bleakest, cancer after cancer.

In closing this chapter I ask you to be heartened by accounts of those tumors that have spread widely and yet have been wiped out, such as the germ cell cancers in young men and women; the rare re-missions of renal cell cancer or malignant melanoma; and the occa-sional patient with advanced disease who responds dramatically to an old drug or a new cancer vaccine. These may be the mysteries of Peregrine the saint, but they tell us that advanced cancers can be controlled if we apply vigorously the sharp and targeted methods of his falcon companion. For the first time since human cancers have been known to the planet, we know where we need to go, and can draw the maps to get us there.

But that's not enough. Great medical advances are driven by public passion and a sense of urgency. Be it polio or heart disease, AIDS or breast cancer, strong public will is paramount to success. On this, the cancer scorecard with its successes and failures speaks for itself.

PART FIVE

Patient Empowered

Not in the clamor of the crowded street,
Not in the shouts and plaudits of the throng,
But in ourselves, are triumph and defeat.

—"The Poets,"
Henry Wadsworth Longfellow

CHAPTER 12

Personal Choice

A CANCER DIAGNOSIS LEAVES you little time to feel sorry for yourself, however much you might be justified in doing so. There is too much to be done, and the world you have just entered calls upon wit and reserves you never knew you had. Even though you want to close your eyes and let someone else take over, you are the one who will live with the decisions made along the way. Your knowledge and choices will play a critical role in your care. Medical information was once a mystery of the temple, its secrets wrapped in obscure language and hidden in journals read only by those in the guild. Now at your fingertips, on the air, and from your computer screen—added to what you hear from your doctors—is information about your condition, ongoing research, and options for care.

Although a cancer diagnosis inspires a sense of urgency, you have places to go, doctors to see, and choices to make. Ordinarily there is time to get smart, however great the pressure might seem to get on with therapy. That cancer of yours has been percolating for a while, and unless it has triggered an acute surgical emergency, such as a bowel obstruction that needs immediate attention, you and your family have some time to take a breath and become informed.

Rules of Engagement

There are some caveats in this world of abundant medical information, however. In what you glean from your own research or in discussions with your doctor, you will find some sharp statistics, a range of options, and complex treatment protocols that can be confusing. Patients have to realize up front that the knowledge base of cancer medicine is about averages of different groups of people who are not always just like them. Few of us are textbook cases. Added to that, from report to report statistics can get fuzzy, if not conflicting. Nonetheless, medicine needs these metrics to follow the natural history of a disease and monitor the success or failure of different treatments. But the averages still reflect bell-shaped curves, and patients would do well to remember this. They are not your destiny. They do not forecast how many weeks you will live or your chance of surviving five years. Never put yourself in the straitjacket of other people's averages.

A friend of mine from high school brought this point home to me. I had not seen her for decades, but we met at a lunch in New York City at which close to half of my Hunter High School class gathered. I'll call her Julia. Some six years earlier, Julia had been diagnosed with stage III endometrial cancer and was told by her doctors that she would be lucky to live eighteen months. Based on that, she retired from a job she loved as a successful executive in a large New York bank. Today she remains cancer free—a cure by any other name. Bored and eager to resume working, she bitterly regrets the retirement. Unfortunately, in her late fifties, her opportunities to jump back into the game at an executive level were virtually gone.

Had her doctors encouraged her to keep working at something she loved despite her illness, she believes, her life would be quite different today. Julia's story is not unusual, and as more people become long-term survivors, it is one to remember. So is that of Stephen Jay Gould.

The late Harvard biologist wrote a now-famous essay about his own confrontation with an abdominal mesothelioma, a rare cancer of the lining of the abdominal cavity. In "The Median Isn't the Message," he argues that no average could or should be applied to any one individual. Once diagnosed with his cancer, Gould asked his doctor where to find out more about his disease (this was pre-Internet). She told him that the "literature contained nothing really worth reading." His own research turned up the reason for her reticence: the disease was "terminal," with a median survival time of eight months from the time of diagnosis. However, as an evolutionary biologist, Gould understood that while statistics have their usefulness, they do not provide the hard and fast answers that most of us think they do. Rather, they provide a set of overall, general guidelines that don't necessarily define any one person's experience.

Gould knew that the median is simply the halfway point in a series. In fact, half of the people diagnosed with this type of cancer would live for *more* than eight months. So he kept on reading to see why. What other factors did these people have in common? He was relieved to discover that, like them, his disease had been caught before it had advanced too far, he wasn't old, and his medical care would be first-rate. There was an additional fact that cheered Gould on: from his familiarity with statistics, he understood that the data for his disease had been skewed in one direction, which meant there was a good chance he'd be alive much longer than those eight months. And he was correct: Gould survived for twenty years after that original diagnosis, and eventually succumbed to a different type of cancer. In those two decades he had a full and highly productive life, published several books, and offered much to his family, his students, and to the world.

Dire predictions and harsh words such as *terminal* are common-place in oncology, yet uncommon in most other medical fields, even when they deal with the very sick. When a patient's heart disease is advanced or he is ready for a transplant, we don't think of his case as being terminal. After all, life is terminal, and the phrase has little meaning except for its chill. There is no ordinary life, and medical crystal balls are not reliable. Of course, it is important to understand what the reality of your situation is in general terms, but be like Stephen Jay Gould, not like my high school friend Julia. Don't let grim words and numbers rule your life. When I was doing research on my tumor, I came across some gruesome numbers much like Gould's, but intuitively I resisted them. Perhaps that's just the tem-perament of an optimist, though I'd rather call it being a realist—why not assume that you're going to be on the right side of any bell-shaped curve that's drawn for you?

Believe me, I did not like my numbers. What helped to order my thinking, however, was that they were all over the place. I could see that my tumor was lumped in with others of a different type, which made it easier for me to dismiss the statistics I didn't like. The only time I ever had a needed negative jolt came early in my hospitaliza-tion. In a conversation with one of my doctors about options that would give me the most quality time, I said, "So, what if I do noth-ing?" Without a pause he responded, "A few months." That state-ment packed a wallop, and I never went there again.

At times like these, it helps to be not only an optimist but also a bit of a philosopher. Think of Pascal's wager. The seventeenth-century French philosopher Blaise Pascal laid out a process for de-ciding which path to take in the face of probable outcomes. Pascal struggled with the ultimate philosophical question: atheism versus theism. As he saw it, faith in God leads to either heaven or hell; athe-ism, however, leads only to hell. So, he concluded, have faith in God. You just might gain everything, and if you are wrong, you lose nothing. If you don't have faith, as Pascal saw it, you face certain damnation, and gain nothing if you are right. Why not apply some version of Pascal's wager to that bell-shaped curve that wraps around every cancer patient? Have faith that you will gain some serious living time. If your wager turns out right, you win doubly; if wrong, you lose nothing. If you believe the opposite, you will spend your days waiting for doom to strike and be robbed of the time you do have.

There's an NBC cameraman whose wager turned out right. I know him as a forthright man with a slight, wiry frame, but I was astonished to discover that his slimness was the result of a major brush with pancreatic cancer more than ten years ago. At the time, his only symptom was back pain. Pancreatic cancer is one of those that bears pretty dismal numbers, and it's easy to find them: a less than 5 percent chance of surviving five years. He was given a few months at most and told to get his affairs in order. A Whipple operation performed at Johns Hopkins saved him. Here he is now, healthy, happy, fully engaged in life, and very proud of his survival. I only learned about it because of an MSNBC interview in which I said that patients often fool you; many a doctor has been humbled by the long life of so-called terminal patients. After the interview, he came over and told me with a big smile that he was one of them. He finds himself encouraging many a friend and colleague as they face cancer. Was his an improbably good outcome? Yes. But had he not remained positive despite the worst of all odds, how miserable his life would have been these many years.

Cancer-speak can be downright toxic. Anybody diagnosed with cancer feels helpless and can be easily intimidated by medical experts. Medical articles can overwhelm with cancer-speak, too. One of my least favorite terms, standard in medical practice and research therapeutics, is *salvage therapy,* which refers to the treatment given to a patient after a relapse when other treatments have failed, like it's a tugboat taking on a wreck. You don't want to promote false hope among the patient and his or her family, of course, but there are words and there are words.

Long before I was in medicine I rebelled against this kind of medicalese. When I was growing up in Queens, we often drove across the 59th Street Bridge to Manhattan. My parents told us about a large, dark building tucked under the bridge on what was then known as Welfare Island that had once been named the Hospital for Incurables. I imagined the terror of being sent to such a place, with so dreary a location and so hateful a name. At one time, however, that was all medicine had to offer—something that today seems unimaginable. Of course, a physician must speak frankly with a patient who has exhausted all of the available therapies, even if the next option is hospice. But most patients know intuitively when the end of their journey is near.

Sometimes, even today, a rigid system and ingrained medical attitudes can keep a patient from taking a wager on life. I have a dear friend, Helen, whose brother was stricken with a brain tumor only a few years after I became ill. After being evaluated at home, he traveled thousands of miles to the Cleveland Clinic for a second opinion, which recommended a course of treatment that made sense to him. He was ready to go—until he returned home, where his oncologist was not pleased. The local doctor would not accept the Cleveland plan or the newer chemo that had been suggested, even though Helen and her husband were quite prepared to cover its cost and ship the drugs to him. The patient was told, in essence, that unless he went with the home team, he would not be cared for, and his health plan proved inflexible. His poor wife became distraught and pressured him to go along. To keep the peace he did so, but until the end, according to his sister, he kept wondering whether things would have turned out better for him had he followed the treatment that brought him the most confidence.

Confident, hopeful patients, undiminished by pompous know-it-all doctors or rigid bureaucratic systems, are part of good cancer care. Doctors have certainly gotten better than they were in the old days, when no one questioned their pontification. And patients need to know that even with rigid doctors or restrictive health insurance plans, there is almost always some give in the system. No patient should be bullied into a treatment, for no one doctor or institution has all the answers.

This brings me to what I think may be the worst of all medical types: the "I am God" doctors, a rare but difficult breed that most of us in the profession know and do not treasure. Often charismatic, hardworking, and very controlling, brimming with received wisdom that they will quickly tell you others lack, such doctors often pile on one toxic treatment after another to the very end, even when common sense says that it will bring no benefit, only more pain and suffering. Patients either love them or butt heads with them. The "I am God" doctors are also the ones who say, in essence, *Do it my way or you die. I'm the one above all who will save you.* I've known a few, and my advice is to avoid them like the plague.

This just might explain the unnecessary and tragic ruckus that occurred in Corpus Christi, Texas, in early 2005. Katie Wernecke, a thirteen-year-old girl with Hodgkin's disease, became the center of a custody battle in large part triggered by her doctor. In short, the thirteen-year-old and her parents declined the oncologist's orders for radiation treatments to her chest at a time when she had had four cycles of chemotherapy, which they were told had put her in remission. The parents were concerned about the risk of early breast cancer, a legitimate concern. The parties battled back and forth over the treatments. Triggered by the doctor's assertion that without his prescribed therapy the girl would die, the state brought in child protection workers, armed with a court order and backed up by a sheriff's posse. They chased down the tearful Katie, took her from her parents and three brothers, and put her in a foster home. During the battle, Katie's cancer recurred. Because of the recurrence her time in foster care stretched into months, and decisions about a new plan of therapy were made by the state agency and her state-assigned physicians, not her parents. Things went from bad to worse when Katie, held in a strange city, away from her family and friends, refused treatments and grew despondent. Finally, after numerous court pleas, a new judge stepped in and rescinded the state's custody, returning Katie to her parents, but in a seriously deteriorated state.

The agency and the doctor may have been well intentioned, and the parents may have seemed difficult in the eyes of both. But it's hard to believe that the state did not commit a major blunder when it ignored the parents' and the young girl's wishes and imposed instead the oncologist's orders, particularly since the medical orders were by no means chiseled in stone, as the court was led to believe. There were other protocols for treating Hodgkin's that substitute more chemo for radiation for those who go into remission, for the very reasons raised by Katie's family. James Nachman, a Hodgkin's researcher and pediatric oncologist at the University of Chicago, told me, "I would not hesitate to bring in Child Services to insist on cancer treatment that parents are resisting if it's a matter of life or death, but radiation for Hodgkin's disease is surely not one of them."

This case should be studied in every medical school and law school in America as an example of exactly how not to offer cancer care. Almost always there is room to work with patients who have certain treatment concerns. The family voiced legitimate and informed questions, and the father told me early on in the dispute that they would have allowed for more chemotherapy as an alternative. But instead they and their daughter got caught up in a bullying medical and legal system that spiraled out of control. This is the kind of medical tyranny that gives Americans chills about any kind of coercive health care system, be it a rigid HMO that limits choice or a government-run system filled with proscriptions and restrictions on care.

This encounter brings to mind another, also involving a young Texan and his concerned parent. The young man came down with advanced testicular cancer and was evaluated by a leading Houston oncologist. The doctor told the patient up front that his was one of the worst cases possible, and the only shot at a good outcome was if he immediately put himself under the care of that oncologist and his medical center for treatment. The doctor is said to have told him:

"I'm going to kill you. Every day, I'm going to kill you, and then I'm going to bring you back to life." He also told the patient that the price for saving his life would be giving up his choice of career: since one of the standard treatments would damage his lungs, the patient had to forget professional sports. The words of the first doctor did not sit well with the patient and his mother, and with her help and that of an Internet-savvy friend, he found a doctor with a different style and a different treatment plan, which made all the difference.

The patient, of course, was Lance Armstrong, before he was rich and famous and the winner of even one Tour de France. The story is recounted in detail in his book *It's Not About the Bike*. There he describes the despair he felt after the conversation with his Houston doctor and his determination to quickly find another opinion. Armstrong and his mom promptly went off to Indianapolis, where experts with a somewhat more humble approach met with him. The Indiana doctors accepted the prior oncologist's advice as standard but suggested that they modify the customary approach so that he could return to bicycle racing. They replaced the lung-scarring drug with another chemo agent. Also, to eliminate risk of problems with mental and physical coordination, they substituted neurosurgery for the more damaging radiation in order to wipe out the two areas of cancer in his brain. As Armstrong relates it, the first doc focused on survival, the second on surviving whole. The first tore him down, the second built him up. At the time, Lance Armstrong was twenty-five years old. It's a good thing he wasn't eight years younger when he fell sick, or he, too, might have been forced into treatment that neither he nor his mother wanted. Had that occurred, his life—and sports history—would never have been the same.

These patients' experiences also point out how doctors sometimes focus more on the grim details of the cancer itself rather than on the side effects of the heavy-duty cancer treatments, often leaving patients unsure about what to expect. Although it still holds true that the sicker the patients, the more vulnerable and compliant they are, gone are the days when patients blindly followed the advice of their physicians. Since it is the patient who must live with the results, it's not wrong to expect care that is sensitive to an individual's life circumstances and personal choices.

Indeed, the most basic of research at the genomic and proteomic level has already shown us the shortfalls, if not folly, of nonpersonalized care. And contrary to the notion that the gene chip and the supercomputer might replace the bedside as the place where medicine is carried out, more than ever we will need smart and commonsensical clinicians to lead the patient through the swamp of new variables, statistics, and bell-shaped curves that will be cut ever so much more finely as we begin to fathom the nature of any one cancer. For it to come out right, personalized treatment must also be a time of evaluating patients in the context of their lives and their dreams. In the wisdom of Sir William Osler, one of the founding doctors of Johns Hopkins Hospital, whose words were etched everywhere during my training there, "From the standpoint of medicine as an art for the prevention and cure of disease, the man who translates the hieroglyphics of science into the plain language of healing is certainly more useful." And healing takes a heap of humility.

Becoming Informed

Unlike most other illnesses where one doctor will generally do, in the course of cancer care you will come to rely on groups of doctors, nurses, and other professionals working together on your behalf. When you are surrounded by a sea of new faces and strange vocabularies, engulfed by high-tech equipment and sometimes overwhelming numbers, deciding which way to go can be an Alice in Wonderland experience. Your way out of the maze is a combination of learning about your own illness and finding a medical team that you trust. You are no prima donna for wanting this.

Lots is written about cancer from the patient's perspective, and generally it makes for comforting reading. And as anyone who has ever typed in something on Google knows, the Internet is a fantastic resource. This does not mean that the information that's out there can't be rough sledding or conflicting. The sheer amount of information can overwhelm you if you're not careful, and it can be frustrating and discouraging if you don't get some medical guidance to make sense of it. One of the best guides is the Web site of the National Cancer Institute. Even its URL is easy: www.cancer.gov. An equally good place to turn is the American Cancer Society, www.cancer.org. These are both reliable and authoritative starting points, very much geared to the information needs of patients and their families. Both are user-friendly portals to gradually orient consumers to the vast sea of cancer information on the Web. You will find yourself returning to them regularly like a trusted friend.

No doubt, being medically trained made it easier for me to sift through whatever information I could find on my relatively rare tumor. But I am always impressed how others—medically trained or not—quickly absorb medical knowledge when their own health is involved. Look at some of the Internet chat rooms out there. Patients bombard each other with endless questions and report on new information as if they were members of a medical journal club.

You can choose almost any tumor type and listen in as the conversation fills the ether. Take, for example, the matter of radiation treatment and Hodgkin's disease, the very issue that led to Katie Wernecke's ordeal. I found one chat room on the topic called "Radiation or Not?" On this site one patient details her remission with six cycles of chemotherapy and says she is just not sure whether she should opt for radiation; her doc is giving her the choice. Another chat voice tells her to do it; he's a five-year survivor but relapsed with chemo alone. Another, called Joe, counters with the point that the only consistent thing he has read is that the overall survival is the same regardless of whether you get combined treatment or chemo alone. Other postings warn that more is not always better when it comes to cancer treatment. One regular named TC summarizes—accurately, I might add—recent findings from the *New England Journal of Medicine* on both survival and late complications from Hodgkin's. Simone's mom says it all: "We are working through this exact question at the moment. Thanks for asking it for me." These informed chats should be eye-opening to doctors and inspiring to other patients. In their serious banter they are smart and empowered and wonderfully honest. In the anonymity of the Internet emerges a sensitive and supportive community of people who bear the unique insight that can only come from having walked in a cancer patient's shoes.

What this also shows is that nowadays everyone can access the same information—and when the stakes are high, information is the greatest treasure. Moreover, patients are participating in their own treatment decisions. Does that mean patients are becoming more questioning or even uppity with their doctors? Perhaps. But good doctors respond positively to that, for it's the sign of a patient who is motivated to do some heavy lifting. And good doctors are firm in their recommendations when evidence is solid, more flexible when it is not.

When I delved into the rather obscure field of neuro-oncology and pondered all sorts of details about my own illness, I did so less as a doctor than as a patient with the autonomy cancer patients have won for themselves over the past thirty years, an autonomy that I had celebrated for years as something that vastly improves the medical culture. Since science moves so quickly, no doctor, no scientist, has all the answers on the best choice for any individual. Years ago women with breast cancer demanded a say, and their activism made treatment choice the medical reality it is today. Now men diagnosed with prostate cancer routinely work with their urologists to sort through the known risks and benefits of many different treatment options. This is pretty much routine for virtually all cancers, if that's what patients want.

I was no different. There were options, confounded by the dilemmas of what we knew and didn't know, and the burden of making a choice that only my family and I would live with. I knew there was no easy way out of this, and no choice was without its tradeoffs, but the balancing of risks and benefits had to be on my terms. On this my doctors were terrific. They did not paint rosy pictures or push me in one direction or the other. The cold facts were laid out; they voiced their opinions soberly and clearly. But I, the amateur in their world, with the support of my husband, had the final say. There was no pulling back on their part—as I know there would have been years ago, for me or any other patient. They offered me respect and dignity at a time of weakness and vulnerability. That is something no patient ever forgets, and something everyone should expect.

Brain Trust

You can't escape the reality of modern cancer care, filled with uncertainties, moving targets, new drugs, emerging research, and diverging paths. Different doctors, heavily steeped in their own specialties—whether surgery, medical oncology, radiation therapy, or some other novel therapeutic approach—bring different views. Often consideration of all three treatments in some combination is in order. Everyone needs a brain trust under these circumstances. The ideal is finding a balanced team and engaging them early in your cancer journey. This is not as difficult as it may seem at first; even in today's world of managed care most plans offer flexibility for those undergoing cancer treatment. In reality, a team of doctors will weigh in on your care anyway; chances are you will have visits with most of them at some point. Sure, it was easier for me and my husband to conceptualize this need, but it's an option that can be set up by any patient if he or she selects an oncologist whose practice is to do so.

Today, brain trusts—outgrowths of multidisciplinary clinics— are becoming a part of the fabric of cancer centers just because of their added value. In fact, many cancer centers use this approach as a selling point. A patient comes in for a consultation and meets with the small group of specialists who would potentially be involved in his or her care. They have already reviewed the case, including the pathology and radiology, and present the diagnosis and treatment options to the patient and family. Sometimes there's a phone conference to bring in other voices, both family members and doctors. Obviously, it's harder to make this happen when doctors are not all working under the same roof or integrated into some kind of group practice. But it can be done, and it is vastly better than finding yourself taking your medical charts from place to place seeking information and often hearing seemingly conflicting views that are hard to reconcile. It's more effective, efficient, and patient-friendly for the docs to come together early on and, if need be, at specified times throughout the course of treatment. I recognize that not all patients want to be part of such a group meeting, and that's okay, too. But if a patient does want to meet or hear from the others on their team and it's not done routinely, just ask. Good places will find a way to accommodate you.

In my experience as doctor and patient, there is nothing like having the experts together early on—with you present—as they hash out options, in part prompted by your questions and perspective. Think of these as business meetings of sorts, a time for practical discussion about where you are, where you want to be, and what's next. In our meetings we went over new approaches, including more targeted radiation treatment or ways to improve local chemotherapy with catheters or implanted chemo wafers. We discussed the pros and cons of the many research protocols under way across the country.

Often the brain trust becomes virtual. Occasionally I spoke by telephone to the neuroradiologist, Dr. Paul Ruggieri, at the Cleveland Clinic. He routinely read my accumulating series of MRI scans, and I considered him a crucial part of my care, as I think he did, too. Pathologists and radiologists are silent members of any cancer care team, as their expertise is pivotal both in early decisions and also along the course of treatment and follow-up.

Despite some differences of opinion, my brain trust almost always came up with a short-term plan with which we were all comfortable. They would often remind me that we could not get ahead of ourselves in the therapy, since there were many uncertainties and each new step was still driven by the level of progress of the last several rounds of treatment. We would lay out a plan and agree, at least until we met again. And this is so for almost all patients as they move along their cancer journey, a journey of faith and facts.

I want to emphasize that brain trusts are not just for doctors who know how to wend their way through the medical maze. All patients should expect this kind of care and seek out institutions that promote accessibility and teamwork. So many of the important innovations in the culture of medical practice have been driven by patient demand. I remember when fathers were banned from delivery rooms, when nurses had to stand when a doctor walked into a room, and when patients feared to ask their doctors a question or to ever say no.

What patients should also know is that a version of the brain trust is part of behind-the-scenes cancer care—though patients are not invited. It's called the tumor board. This is a formal mechanism, mandated for accredited hospitals, in which the larger cancer team assembles as a group to discuss individual patients and monitor them through their ups and downs as they move through therapy. These days, tumor boards are organized according to type of cancer, and meet at least weekly. As many as fifty people might be in one room—surgeons, medical oncologists, radiation therapists, pathologists, radiologists, oncology nurses, nutritionists, geneticists, and clinical and sometimes basic researchers. Think of these meetings as a kind of grand rounds, except they are not primarily for teaching. Rather, they are working sessions directed at individual patient care. Tough cases get more extensive discussion. New ideas surface, complications are reviewed, and progress is tracked. This offers an extra level of oversight and expertise. Knowing that other experts are vetting your case should be a comfort and offers you the chance to ask your oncologist about their discussions. Question your doctor about the points of agreement or disagreement that may have come up. You are the topic, and you have every right to know the gist of their deliberations.

Weighing in with your own personal choice is no easy task. It takes time and engagement and invariably is fraught with frustration and unease. Some doctors, quite frankly, are not keen about patients knowing too much or asking too many questions. That's all the more reason to choose doctors and medical centers that fit with your own temperament—and, as I detail in the next chapter, to tap into some novel sources to help guide you on this journey of a lifetime.

CHAPTER 13

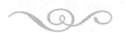

Medics, Mentors, and Cancer Centers

ANCER HOSPITALS HAVE BEEN with us for over a hundred years, but the notion of designated cancer centers with an integrated system of care is one that has emerged in response to the demands of modern-day integrated therapy. Today's cancer center is home to cross-specialty activity focusing on patient care, education, and research for cancers of all kinds, and rendering both short- and long-term care. All disciplines of medicine are represented, along with other specialized functions, such as nutrition, pain therapy, hospice and home care, and social and family support services.

The notion of an integrated and accredited cancer program reflected in today's cancer center has its roots in the work of the American College of Surgeons (ACS), which in 1922 established a multidisciplinary Commission on Cancer to set formal standards for quality cancer care in what was then almost exclusively the hospital setting. Very much ahead of its time, the group has fostered uniform organizational requirements, including education, clinical research, quality assurance programs, and enhanced patient and family services. By ACS standards, accredited cancer centers must have tumor registries that record and track all cancer patients and provide the information to state and federal data banks, as well as meet other standards of patient care, such as the tumor boards mentioned earlier.

Cancer centers have become national resources, providing a powerful network of care throughout the country. These institutions work together in their research and educational efforts and participate in an extensive system of multicenter clinical trials. For almost any patient's cancer there is likely to be a clinical trial exploring a new therapy. Joanne Hilden, the head of pediatric oncology at the Taussig Cancer Center, is proud to tell you that 80 percent of pediatric patients nationally enroll in clinical trials, where they receive great overall care, as well as the latest in treatments.

There are about 9,000 new cases of pediatric cancer a year. Since they are such rare events and fit into a narrow category of disease types, most children with cancer receive care from specialty centers that customarily are part of NIH-sponsored clinical trial networks. Compare this to the hundreds of different cancers that arise each year in adults; there are not enough trials for them all. And trials are not for everyone. Patients have to meet certain eligibility requirements; and some patients don't want to give up their choice of therapy. Others are concerned that they might get a toxic drug that won't work, or mistakenly think they might get a placebo when other people are getting the good stuff. This, by the way, is not the case, as the drugs studied in the large patient trials have already been tested for safety and side effects. And in cancer trials, no patient is given placebo therapy.

The important thing to know is that clinical trials are available to most patients who want to be part of them, depending mainly on their geographic location. Currently, the National Cancer Institute has a list of more than 2,000 trials that are actively enrolling patients; they are described on the NCI Web site. (See pages 228–230 for more information.)

Entering a clinical trial can be an opportunity for patients to get access to the latest therapy in an environment that is immersed in the cutting-edge developments of the field. But patients need to learn about the trial, become comfortable with its structure and the follow-up demands it makes on their person or time, and of course understand its risks. Strict ethical guidelines ensure the patient's informed consent and also allow for patients to drop out of a trial if they wish to do so for any reason and at any point; the center is still obliged to continue with their care. Patients should know that they do not get free care because they participate in a trial, but they do get the drug being tested at no cost, as well as any research-related additional care.

With their tumor registries and clinical trial networks, cancer centers have become important repositories of nationwide research and information. Over time certain centers develop a particular expertise with one form of cancer, usually based on their research work. Johns Hopkins is world famous for its work in colon cancer, Stanford is known for lymphoma research, Northwestern has had a major program in breast cancer prevention and treatment, and St. Jude's Hospital for Children in Memphis is renowned for its work on childhood cancers. But most designated cancer centers have expertise with most cancers and hold to a high level of overall patient care. Patients who are willing to travel can be seen at almost any of them, and for the most part these centers cooperate and communicate effectively. It's not at all uncommon for a treatment plan to be devised in one center and carried out in another. With the right doctors and the right health plan, cooperation happens seamlessly. Good doctors consult one another, and those at specialty centers regularly work with local oncologists. Patients understandably cling to home when they are seriously ill. They want to be near family, friends, and familiar faces, not to speak of the financial cost and

emotional strain of undergoing extended treatment in a distant city.
(The exception might be for specific procedures, such as a new technology or surgical expertise with a particular operation.)

For me, the Cleveland Clinic was my place. Sure, there were
other institutions in the country that had fancier names or were
ranked higher nationally by *U.S. News & World Report*. But I was confident in the Taussig Cancer Center and its presence in the obscure
world of brain tumors, and I felt at home with my early dealings
with my brain trust. Though I'd considered other suggestions for
care, which kindly came in from many of my friends and colleagues
elsewhere, I had no doubts about staying put. I can assure you that if
I'd had any qualms, I would have been gone in a flash. But once
you're satisfied with the quality, there is something to be said for
comfort, convenience, and familiarity. Chances are you'll be working with your chosen doctors and their institution for a long time, so
you want to make it a thoughtful choice. Ultimately, the impressive
buildings and the high-powered Web sites don't take care of you—
it's the doctors and nurses who do. If you find the right ones—and
there are plenty out there—they will help guide you through this
complex and often arduous experience.

⁓ FINDING CANCER CARE ⁓

How can you find a cancer center that's not only first-rate but
skilled in caring for your type of tumor? Start in your own back-
yard. There are excellent cancer centers throughout the country,
and with a little checking from friends, neighbors, and your own
medical network, you can find out about the reputation of centers
in your own locality. Be sure they have the talent and the technology that is needed for your particular problem; today that includes access to strong pathology and genetics departments. Most
centers have these resources, but it does not hurt to ask questions:
Will your biopsy be reviewed by this or another center, particu-

larly if there is some uncertainty about it? Are there newer genetic tests, there or elsewhere, that might help sort out the nature of your disease?

In addition to talking to your physician and other personal sources, there are a number of excellent resources available to you as well. *U.S. News & World Report* annually ranks the top cancer centers in the country (click on "Best Hospitals" on www.usnews.com). The rankings are based on a mix of peer specialist evaluation, facilities and resources offered to the patient, and patient outcome. For other centers near you, contact the local chapter of the American Cancer Society (www.cancer.org). Or ask around for the name of a good oncology nurse; they are on the front lines in the battle against cancer.

For information about specific cancers, the Web site of the National Cancer Institute (www.cancer.gov) is tops, with reliable and easily accessible information regarding the different types of tumors. If you click through the NCI site, you will find lists of the cancer programs and centers it funds across the country and descriptions of the many clinical trials it sponsors, which usually includes the names and contact numbers of those working in the field you are interested in.

The National Library of Medicine, the largest medical library in the world, has a terrific service (www.pubmed.gov) that can provide you with summaries of scientific studies regarding your specific tumor. You can type in "breast cancer," for example, and see abstracts for all of the relevant peer-reviewed journal articles. While some of this information is highly technical, it will give you a good idea of the kinds of research that is happening, who is doing it, and at which institutions.

The National Library of Medicine also hosts a Web site (www.clinicaltrials.gov) that in a click informs doctors and their patients of clinical trials that might be of value to them. Even if you do not want to enter a specific trial, it is worth reviewing the clinical trials to find out about the latest work that is going on, and the list provides names and contact numbers should you want to be in touch with the institutions directly. Additionally, many drug companies sponsor trials of their new drugs, which can be accessed through these same individuals and institutions or by going on the Web site of the company that manufactures the drug or device.

The Best Doctor for You

We all want good doctors when staring down a serious illness. Figuring out whom to turn to is made a lot easier if you have an established relationship with an internist or other physician who can advise you and ideally stay involved along the way. You should go into the process with high expectations for your cancer specialists. Cancer care calls for doctors who are smart and up-to-date; in a field that is evolving so rapidly, they should be scholarly, thoughtful, and independent in processing the raft of new studies appearing almost daily. You also want professionals guided by common sense, which is a big part of good medical care.

But finding the right doctor and not stopping until you are satisfied with the combination of medical and human skills does sometimes mean seeking out another opinion. In fact, most hospitals help patients find cancer specialists, and if one doctor or clinic does not seem to fit, there is no shame in looking further. It's only a shame if you don't. Sometimes a particular doctor may make you feel uncomfortable; the chemistry just doesn't seem right. Perhaps you don't like the doctor's attitude, or feel as if your questions are being disregarded or demeaned. Don't be afraid to look elsewhere, the sooner the better. Even if you are already into therapy, another opinion or even another doctor can be the right thing to do. Don't worry about offending anyone or burning any bridges. A doctor may be just right for the friend or colleague who gave you the referral and may be highly qualified, held in high esteem, and in great demand, but if it's not a good match for you, move on.

What will emerge from the process is a leader of your cancer team with whom you are comfortable. The lead doctor is also determined by the kind of tumor you have and the primary type of treatment. For example, a medical oncologist leads in breast cancer care, a hematology-oncology specialist in leukemia and lymphoma treatment, and a surgeon or radiotherapist for cases of prostate or head and neck cancer.

Beyond being comfortable with and trusting your physician as a person, you must know about his or her skill and experience. If you are going to come under the knife, find out how many procedures similar to yours that individual surgeon has performed in the past year, and the resulting complications rate. The same holds for a bone marrow transplant. Doctors and hospitals keep track of this information, but you usually have to ask.

I have a good friend, a smart businesswoman from New York, who called me regarding her husband's planned surgery for early prostate cancer. His general urologist was set to do a radical prostatectomy. I encouraged her to find out exactly how many of these he did a year, and rather than relying on published statistics on bleeding, infection, long-term incontinence, or impotence, I suggested she ask what this particular surgeon's own numbers looked like. It turned out that his annual experience was small and his outcomes were not as good as those reported in the literature. The couple promptly went to Memorial Sloan-Kettering for a second opinion and found a more experienced surgeon.

Does that mean the outcome would have been different had my friend's husband stayed with his general urologist? Not necessarily. But he definitely improved his odds. Time and time again, physicians and hospitals that do a lot of a certain procedure perform better, and their short- and long-term results show it. Just recently, in a study in the *Journal of Clinical Oncology*, researchers at Virginia Commonwealth University showed that, especially for complicated cancer surgery, patients were better off, as measured by five-year survival rates, when they went to medical institutions that were high-volume, rather than institutions that were known mainly for their cancer research. (These, by the way, are not mutually exclusive.) Experience matters in most things; why should it not in medical care? To get these numbers, all you have to do is ask.

Oncology Nurses

In the process of finding the right doctors, you will discover the people who are often the unsung experts of cancer care: oncology nurses. They are active and informed members of your cancer team, ready to answer questions, administer therapies, and oversee complex treatment schedules. These highly skilled professionals are also frequently the ones who are there to listen to your fears and concerns and to offer encouragement and emotional support. They may be your principal guides through the different steps of treatment and the first to greet you when you return for follow-up care. Most cancer patients can regale you with stories about the special kindnesses of their oncology nurses. Just after my surgery, I met with one of the oncology nurses in the Brain Tumor Institute who introduced me to my new world with the thick folder of information given to all initiates. This cancer stuff was new to me, and she was the sure-footed expert. I heard about wound care and diet, support groups and lectures. At one point we locked glances and her eyes briefly welled up as she saw me barely listening to her, silently struggling and distracted. That brief glance from a tender heart gave me more comfort than any of her words.

Another time, a nurse came to the dressing room after a procedure to help me get my stuff together. She told me about her sister, who was struggling with a breast cancer recurrence. A devout Christian, she asked me if I would like to hold her hand as she prayed—for both of us. Her offer was not in any way intrusive; it was a sincere touch of a tender woman who saw this as a form of healing, too, and I accepted it. Whether in emergency rooms, recovery rooms, intensive care units, or outpatient clinics, the good nurses whom I have worked with during my years in medicine—as doctor and as patient—are the lifeblood of the hospital.

Maureen Bell, an Irish Catholic from a big Cleveland family, became my principal oncology nurse; even now I see her during my routine follow-up visits. Her crisp, cheerful efficiency has not changed one iota. However grim things looked for me early on, she was always smiling, never making promises but always offering hope. I recall when she became pregnant and I wondered whether I would ever see her child. Now each time I see her she shows me yet another photo of her sprouting young son. When I accepted the job at the American Red Cross, which meant being in Washington during the week, she assured me she would be at the Taussig on the Fridays when I came in from the airport for my counts and blood port care—for, despite the new job, I still had months of chemotherapy ahead of me. One day I came home to our Washington apartment and found in my mail a Celtic stone cross from Maureen, intended to watch over me there. It hangs in our entry hall, on the wall adjacent to a sepia print of a World War I Red Cross nurse. (In those days the Red Cross ran a nursing school and provided all the nurses for the war.) In the print, whose original hangs in the Red Cross Museum, a young nurse in her white apron and blue cape is cradling in one arm a wounded soldier on the battlefield; her other arm is outstretched as she fends off a large and threatening image of the Grim Reaper lurking over her shoulder. I never consciously connected Maureen's cross with this print, but both capture the spirit of the nurse.

There are numerous other good souls who work in cancer care—from the ward assistants, nutritionists, and MRI techs to the rehab folks and palliative care workers. Those who gravitate to this trying field recognize intuitively that what a cancer patient craves above all is to be in the hands of experts who are also trusted and caring souls. We have common wants: doctors and nurses and other health care workers who explain what is going on, are there with round-the-clock ministrations if need be, and at the same time respect their patients' autonomy and honor their decisions.

Mentors

In the olden days of medicine, it was said you could cure half the sick by putting them into bed and the other half by getting them up. And the doctor always knew which was which, for he (almost always a he) had very few options in his little black bag. Medical decisions followed a straight course. Not anymore. We are increasingly the beneficiaries of a medical world that knows more and can do more. For almost any illness, including cancer, the paths to be taken are more maze than unbending line. Today doctors may present options and offer preferences, but ultimately it's the patient's decision which course to follow. I recognize that this is easier said than done. It's hard to feel empowered to make those decisions if you aren't sure which way to go. In fact, several medical studies have shown that many people faced with important medical decisions wished they'd had more help even in framing the right questions to ask their doctors, not to mention weighing the risks and benefits of several types of therapy. Patients should never hesitiate, by the way, to ask their doctor, "What would you do if you were me, and why?" That's really the ultimate question. Most doctors will be frank with you.

Fred Rogers, the late and beloved children's television personality, related how, when he was a child, his mother would counsel him, "Look for the helpers. You will always find people who are helping." I can't think of better advice to give anyone facing a cancer journey. One kind of helper is what I call the medical mentor. Mentors or guides can help you find the doctor or cancer care center that's right for you. They can help you negotiate with a tyrannical specialist, help by being a sounding board for any number of crucial decisions regarding your treatment and care, or be a source of informed support during the up times and the down times alike.

In short, *mentor* seems to be the best word to describe those special people who are often the hidden guides for patients moving through the cancer odyssey.

Mentors do odysseys. In Greek mythology, it was the wizened old Mentor who guided Telemachus, the son of Odysseus, as he set off in search of his father. Mentor was an in-the-background kind of guy, but he was always there to help with fateful choices. Were that not enough, Mentor had an additional dimension: he was none other than Athena, the goddess of wisdom, who took on the form of Mentor just to help Telemachus. That image informs a modern-day medical mentor—wise, experienced, trusted, available, unobtrusive, and coming in any shape or form. Every bit as important, a mentor takes on this role out of human kindness and not for personal gain. In a biblical sense, mentoring is a mitzvah, a good deed that is its own reward.

A few years ago in an article for *U.S. News & World Report*, as part of a series on "smart patients," I wrote about Cindy Sweeting, a high-powered executive and mother of two who was hit with breast cancer in her mid-forties. From the beginning, she treated her illness as a journey to a place she had never been before, and one that needed the right guides. "I cannot imagine planning a trip for your life where you don't have a guide who has seen it with their own eyes, or maybe even lived there before," she told me. Having worked in the investment banking field for years, she was comfortable making lots of decisions, but was admittedly sometimes overwhelmed by the many choices she had to make in a short time frame. Which doctors to see? Lumpectomy or mastectomy? Yes or no to breast reconstruction? Reading can only get you so far. Though a private person, she actively sought out medically knowledgeable mentors to help—some friends, some she'd never met before—who provided perspective that was relevant to her own personal circumstances. She wanted three things in her guides: experience, knowledge, and trustworthiness.

The first and most obvious person was her close college friend

Suzanne Grimes. She and Suzie both had children, close families, and high-octane jobs, and both were hit with breast cancer at a relatively young age. Cindy had admired her friend's courage and decisiveness when she went through cancer; that was how she wanted to handle her own illness. When Cindy's first biopsy was negative but she was still uneasy about the lump she could feel, Suzie strongly encouraged her to insist on another biopsy. And when the second biopsy was positive, Suzie was there, calm, positive, offering tips on hair and clothes, translating doctor-speak, and giving her positive encouragement about how she could balance treatment cycles with her work and home life.

There were other guides, too. Cindy called on a close friend of her late mother, Jane Pfeiffer, to help her with the task of finding the right doctors, preferably close to home. Jane, whom I've known for years, is a softly plainspoken, ever so kind, and deeply religious woman who is full of common sense. She had had her own bout with cancer years before, and had lost her husband to the disease. Through Jane's experience at the Mayo Clinic, and a few conversations with some of her friends, she found a medical team near where Cindy lived and worked.

But as Cindy points out, mentors need not be people you already know. Cindy thought long and hard about breast reconstruction. In a casual conversation she had with her real-estate agent, he happened to mention that his wife was a veteran of breast cancer and was part of a local neighborhood group of about forty women who had also been there. Though not at all used to having personal discussions with neighbors or perfect strangers, she called the agent's wife to find a woman in her community who had had the procedure. Through that source she met Betsy, who arrived at Cindy's home laden with food and a bottle of wine, chatted with her for quite some time, and then showed Cindy just what her own reconstruction looked like. This meeting became critical to Cindy's decision and brought added comfort to her final choice.

Mentors are a special breed; it's not a job for everyone. One can be loving and attentive and still be wholly unsuited to mentoring. It calls for a kind of detachment, demanding that mentors keep their own interests and emotions in check. Depending on their temperament and expertise, a spouse or other family member might fill the role beautifully. But sometimes even the most loving family members may need guides themselves and feel uncomfortable in that role. A key point here is that whatever the background, whatever the relationship, know-it-alls need not apply: mentors are guides and not there to control or make decisions on behalf of the patient. They help lay out the specs of the journey and weigh its risks and rewards. Sometimes it's just a matter of being there, of being available.

How can you find someone like that, someone with qualities so singular and special? Most times, such a person is already part of your life, if you only ask. Given what's at stake, people are usually only too willing to help. And they don't have to live nearby; there's always the phone or e-mail. There are formal or informal groups to be tapped, too—good neighbors, a community center, your religious congregation. The mentor may be someone who had a similar illness, a nurse or doctor, or someone schooled in health matters. Mostly it's someone you value and trust.

Complementary Medicine

I'm not at all surprised that patients with cancer are major consumers of complementary medicine. After all, it is one domain of therapy that is driven by personal choice, something patients want when they are sick. And increasingly, as complementary medicine has gained more respect by mainstream medicine, its use has become more accepted and widespread.

Back in 1992, when I was at NIH, we began the Center for Complementary Medicine, without a whole lot of enthusiasm from the medical research community. In fact, it was Tom Harkin, senator from Iowa and then chair of the powerful Appropriations Committee, which doled out our annual budget, who made it happen. Harkin was sold on bee pollen for his allergies and was irritated that NIH didn't pay much heed to such remedies or the many others that some 35 to 40 percent of all Americans used regularly.

Without the NIH imprimatur and its financial clout, these remedies would never see respectable daylight. He was right: the mainstream medical literature is now replete with studies of alternative and complementary medicine—and in 1998, Congress christened the effort the National Center for Complementary and Alternative Medicine with a budget in excess of $100 million.

Cancer patients are avid CAM consumers. Even those who never thought twice about things that to some can smack of New Age stuff find themselves using alternative therapies during their cancer journey. Unexplained and unanticipated symptoms for which medicine has no cure prompt many people to try such remedies. Others come to CAM with the complaint that they feel abandoned by their doctors if the medically recommended therapy fails.

This, says Harvard oncologist and essayist Jerome Groopman, may be a valid criticism. Sometimes patients develop a schism with their doctors, and a lot of it, he believes, has to do with the emotional fabric of the caregivers. "Some are remote, statistics-driven, offering patients a jumble of numbers but with little effort to figure out their beliefs, their needs, their goals." He believes that prompts cancer patients to turn to alternative healers. The patients value their doctors but become fed up with the numbers; they want someone who is going to sit with them and focus on their whole being. Cancer treatment is about more than the demise of a tumor; it's also about the physical and emotional effects of a long cancer journey.

For example, one of the biggest surprises about the cancer trek is the bone-crushing fatigue that sets in along the way, mostly as a side effect of treatment. My dear friend Vic Fazio, chairman of colorectal sugery at the Cleveland Clinic, had his tussle with leukemia a few years after I faced cancer. We occasionally compare notes. Both of us are high-energy types who were stunned at how the cancer treatments depleted our energy levels. He noted that no intense, round-the-clock surgery schedule ever caused the same kind of fatigue. We recalled the many days of returning home after putting up a good front at work and dissolving into a puddle of tiredness, barely making it to the nearest chair. Vic's response, with the encouragement of his oncologist, was exercise—a nontraditional form of therapy by historical standards (though one that will never raise eyebrows). Within a few days of leaving the hospital after a bone marrow transplant, he was walking six miles a day.

My somewhat joking response was that I chose the more sedentary route: guided imagery of dying cancer cells, reading my psalms, and—though I have not seen it on anyone's alternative-medicine list—chocolate-glazed donuts. They never failed to give me the lift I needed, at least for a while. And chocolate is just now being seen as a health food—of sorts. Seriously, exercise is important for cancer patients, but so is the urge to find ways, often by trial and error, to feel better, and just maybe discourage the cancer, too.

To be sure, cancer and its treatment threaten both mind and body and bring on a near-primal urge to respond personally to what seems to be out of whack in one's whole system. Most patients turn to alternative medicine to nourish a self under siege. Let their doctors do what they can to destroy the tumor—the patients' quest is for what they can do to fend off the treatment's many side effects and build up their own internal reserves of cancer-fighting abilities, and in the process cope with the psychological pain of the illness. As my friend Vic puts it in his blunt Australian way, it involves dealing with the "uncertainty bit that hovers in the back of your mind."

From massage to acupuncture, yoga to Chinese medicine, chiropractic manipulation to reflexology, music, art, hypnotherapy, and nutritional supplements, these approaches (and many others) are sought out by individuals of varying backgrounds and needs. One study from the Stanford Prevention Research Center found that these therapies in general are used mostly by people who are well educated, who are in the midst of major health problems, and who possess a strong belief in the importance of holistic healing.

The more serious the cancer illness and debilitating the treatment, the more people look to self-healing. Though it was initially thought that people might seek out these types of treatments because they were unhappy with traditional care or because traditional care seemed to have abandoned them, this turns out not to be the case most of the time: people use mainstream and alternative therapies in tandem, and pursue the latter because they fit with their overall attitude and approach toward life. By taking a more active role in their journey to wellness, these patients gain some measure of control over their illness.

To that extent, the choice of complementary therapies, if used at all, is personal and based on whatever works for you. Healing arts, such as guided imagery, massage therapy, yoga, or meditation, can relieve pain, stress, and suffering, bring solace, and perhaps do even more. Acupuncture can help ease the pain of surgery as well as the nausea and vomiting that can be an unwelcome by-product of chemotherapy treatments. For some patients, hypnosis can ameliorate cancer pain as well as the discomfort and anxiety caused by undergoing various procedures, such as bone marrow aspirations, that are a part of the cancer experience.

While I'm bullish on complementary treatments as a personal choice, I have a few strong caveats. For starters, they should never take the place of conventional medical therapy, and your doctor should know what you're doing. Studies indicate that patients often fail to share this information—perhaps out of fear of disapproval. This can create problems, especially if the treatment is ingested, as is the case with dietary supplements, herbs, or other remedies sold in pharmacies and health food stores. I'm the first to admit that nature is loaded with chemicals that have cancer-fighting abilities. The needles of some yew bushes—like the withering ones outside our windows that the pesky deer boldly chomp on—brought us the novel chemotherapy agent Taxol (paclitaxel) not long ago. And chemicals from shark cartilage and the skin of bottom-dwelling sea cucumbers have shown natural abilities to take on certain cancer cells in the laboratory. But as yet, we know little about just what they might do to a human, sick or well. As frustrating as it is that there are many such compounds that are out there aching to be studied, they lack the resources that back newly synthesized and patented drugs. This is just the way it is.

So heed a simple warning: before you start taking any megavitamin, herbal remedy, or folk potion, talk to your doctor. What you're ingesting may be "natural," but many herbs contain strong ingredients, some of which may have their own side effects, or interfere with other drugs that your doctor has prescribed. Another issue is that all too often we just don't know what is the right (if it's right at all) or safe dose to take. High doses of vitamin E, for example, affect platelets and decrease blood clotting, which can be treacherous for a patient who is about to have major surgery or has a low platelet count from chemotherapy. And recently, researchers from Yale have shown that the herb black cohosh, commonly taken to ease the discomforts of menstruation and menopause, interferes with conventional drugs given to breast cancer patients. Before you buy in, do your homework and talk to your medical team.

The Uncertainty Bit

Even with a well-assembled brain trust, a host of mentors, a loving, supportive family, and reams of information on present and future therapies, the cancer journey is a lonely one. At the quiet times the mind has a way of wandering back to the same questions: *What's in store for me? What can I look forward to?* What Vic Fazio calls the "uncertainty bit" is always in the back of your mind. This can be difficult to accept since medicine does vastly better in predicting outcomes for most other illnesses.

For many of us, the operative phrase is "quality of life." We use these words all the time, but you may find that quality of life varies depending on the circumstances in which you find yourself. What at first might seem like a terrible fate may in fact turn out to be not so bad, considering the alternative. Anyone who undergoes the cancer journey comes out with a changed sense of what that quality might be. To me it comes down to this: can you love and can you work? By that I don't necessarily mean paid work, but more the work of every-day living. Love and work are the wellsprings of physical and mental health. If we can operate in these two arenas, we are blessed.

A woman is not happy about having to undergo a mastectomy, but if it contains the cancer and gives her back her life, then it's an easy choice. But if a certain treatment keeps you debilitated, in the hospital, away from loved ones, with the hope of only a few more weeks or months of life, that may be a different matter. Almost thirty years ago, when my dad was dying of lung cancer, his body riddled with tumors despite major surgery and months of radiation and chemotherapy, his blood oxygen levels kept dwindling due to the tumors' infiltrating his lungs and choking off his air passages. Toward the end, one doctor said we might consider a tracheotomy—perhaps it would give him a few more weeks of time. Mom and I had no prob-lem saying no to that. But more important, that would have been Dad's choice, too. I have always been humbled by how very smart our patients can be in such circumstances.

I believe that's one reason why Pope John Paul II's final weeks cap-tured the world's attention. The pontiff made his views crystal clear through his many teachings, which were as much religious as they were common sense and humane: doctors are not "lords of life" but "skilled and generous servants" caring for the sick and dying, offering treatments to cure their patients if possible but always enabling them to bear their sufferings with ease and dignity. He preached that doc-tors should not embark on futile treatments or extraordinary mea-sures when death is imminent and inevitable. But at the same time they should not hasten death. To him a good death was one in the comfort of family, doctors and nurses, and loving friends.

He lived his words. The eighty-four-year-old Holy Father made his choices as his health rapidly declined. He accepted antibiotics, a feeding tube, and two hospitalizations over his last five weeks, but as things grew bleaker, he rejected being moved to the intensive care unit, and having a kidney dialysis or organ resuscitation. Without these, his life faded softly to a final amen. And, perhaps with a wink, he lasted for a time well beyond what Vatican doctors had predicted. Only heaven knows the moment of birthing and dying, the eternal bookends of all our lives. Though in our last moments it is unlikely control will be in our hands, it's more likely that our wishes will be honored if we've had clear and open discussions with those who are caring for us. This is the choice of an empowered patient.

PART SIX

Survivors Rising

Let joy kill you!
Keep away from the little deaths.

—"Joy,"
Carl Sandburg

CHAPTER 14

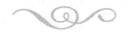

Reaching Out

LINGERING IN MY HEART is a tender note that came to me from a Johns Hopkins colleague early in my illness. She lives with a serious heart condition and has survived deadly rhythms and a cardiac arrest. She wrote: "All of the odds have been stacked against my survival, even worse, against my survival with everything intact. But here I am writing yet another grant, going to work, visiting my daughter in Western Samoa five thousand miles from good medical care. I have learned to approach each day as a gift, although at first that was quite difficult. I've come to realize what incredible courage it takes to go through a serious illness."

Courage is a word we usually associate with wartime. Looking at the cancer experience in terms of what it might teach us about ourselves, of really taking stock, does bring to mind the ceremonies that take place every year on the anniversary of D-Day, June 5. Veterans gather together, revisit their memories or the sites of their battles, and reminisce about the times they shared, both the good and the bad. They remember those who have fallen, and they rejoice in life. That is the attitude of most cancer survivors.

From the children who have battled cancer to the grandparents who have outlasted their tumors, we are here and we are well. Thirty years ago, there were only 3 million cancer survivors alive in the United States. Today, we're nearly 10 million strong and growing in number; we are nearly 3 percent of the population. People who have faced this diagnosis are living longer, and for many of them cancer is a distant memory.

Or is it? Distant and unspoken, perhaps, but the journey is never entirely dimmed by time. As cancer has been transformed from a fatal disease into one that's either cured or chronic, our language has had to change as well, starting with the common moniker *cancer victims*, which carries a sense of helplessness and pathos. We usually know our continued being is due to more than a miraculous intercession similar to what was experienced by St. Peregrine seven centuries ago—even if we cannot nail down with precision the means whereby it happened. Now we are known as *cancer survivors*—a consequential state of being, if one looks closer.

Cancer survivors have experienced life in a very cold and dark place and returned to the light. Yes, we may carry with us a few physical or psychological scars, but overall we're hardier by virtue of just how far we've walked and just how much we've learned. It brings to mind the blackberry winter, a term maybe best known as the title of Margaret Mead's autobiography. This is a time of bitter frost that nips the blackberry's blossom but brings forth a sturdier fruit.

We've all been inspired by the stories of people who retained a positive outlook while staring down their own long, sometimes uncertain blackberry winter, emerging strong and sturdy on their road to wellness. One of the people who's become a legend among cancer survivors is Lance Armstrong, with his record seven consecutive wins of the Tour de France. His accomplishments are all the more incredible because his athletic triumphs were part of his comeback after enduring debilitating treatments for a cancer that had spread to his lungs and his brain by the time it was discovered. Each time he cycled into Paris wearing the leader's yellow jersey and waving the American flag on his final victory lap along the Champs-Elysées toward the Arc de Triomphe, Armstrong did so as the new image of the cancer survivor and an inspiration to every person anywhere in the world who had even a tiny sense of what he had experienced. He has memorialized his triumphs in sports and health through his nonprofit Lance Armstrong Foundation, dedicated to cancer survivors. "Livestrong" is more than a survivors' rallying cry; over 55 million of the ubiquitous yellow bracelets emblazoned with this phrase have been purchased by the citizens of this country and around the world. Not only did they become the latest must-have accessory (and started a fad that has caught on with kids of all ages from coast to coast), but they've increased awareness about many different forms of cancer as well as raised money for cancer research, advocacy, education, and public health.

Armstrong is not the only well-known person to use his fame to educate others about living well and strong beyond cancer and to raise money to further that cause. There's a long list of politicians, athletes, and celebrities who have done the same because they've been touched by the disease in some way. And we know how effective the use of celebrity can be. Katie Couric co-founded the National Colorectal Cancer Research Alliance after she lost her husband, Jay Monahan, at the age of forty-two to the disease. In her mourning she spoke out publicly about the colon cancer that took his life prematurely, and she had a widely covered colonoscopy live on the *Today* show. In the wake of her efforts, the number of colonoscopies performed nationwide increased by 20 percent for almost twelve months. Researchers called it "the Katie Couric effect."

But you don't have to be a celebrity to make a difference. Think of Helga Sandburg Crile, who lives quietly in Cleveland tending her garden and writing poetry. More than thirty years ago she was a pioneer patient, having her early invasive breast cancer picked up by a mammogram—not a common screening test back then. Also ahead of her time, she underwent the equivalent of a lumpectomy, because she had faith that her own pioneering husband, the surgeon George Crile Jr. (Barney to her), was right about tissue-sparing cancer surgery. Helga, now a widow, is a kind and generous woman who reached out to me on many occasions to offer encouragement and show me what it was like to be a joyful survivor. One of her little secrets was that when faced with her own cancer problem she kept replaying in her mind the words of one of her father's earliest poems, which she knew by heart. Carl Sandburg penned "Joy" in 1916:

> *Let a joy keep you.*
> *Reach out your hands*
> *And take it when it runs by . . .*
> *Joy always,*
> *Joy everywhere—*
> *Let joy kill you!*
> *Keep away from the little deaths.*

Cancer survivors are all around us, each with a unique story to tell, and most of them are willing and ready to reach out to others who enter their universe. In 1997, soon after giving birth to her third child, Judy Pickett was diagnosed with breast cancer. She was thirty-three. Since then, she has had two other bouts of the disease and has undergone various rounds of surgery and chemotherapy. But that hasn't stopped this former schoolteacher from running, as part of her Pink Ribbon Running Club, in over a hundred races to benefit the breast cancer cause. All told, she's run with over 2 million people and 100,000 breast cancer survivors. Office Max has sponsored her efforts for a number of years.

About twenty years ago, cancer survivor Richard Bloch, along with his wife, created a media event in Kansas City to highlight the fact that a cancer diagnosis didn't equal certain death, as was the prevailing myth back then. Ever since then, people in hundreds of cities across the country gather on the first Sunday in June to celebrate National Cancer Survivors Day and take part in this joyous, life-affirming celebration. The magazine *Coping with Cancer* has sponsored this effort. Bloch, the co-founder of H & R Block, has since died, but what a legacy he's created for other survivors, who carry on his efforts in one of the largest cancer survivor events each year. In addition, the R. A. Bloch Cancer Foundation supports many educational initiatives, including an informative Web site and a cancer hotline.

There are other ways that survivors reach out to those who are now facing their own cancer trials. They volunteer in hospitals and clinics where treatment or follow-up care is given; they staff hotlines and run support groups and online chat groups; they act as mentors, share information regarding community resources and treatment options, and offer suggestions on how to deal with the less-than-desirable side effects of certain treatments. In the process, survivors have created in effect a *knowledge* movement, working to educate others about their disease and how to advocate for what they need. With that information, better decisions can be made regarding treatment and care.

I am also reminded of Evelyn Lauder, an early activist in the breast cancer awareness effort who was one of the forces behind the first pink ribbon campaign—the ribbon that is now widely recognized as a symbol for living strong against this disease. Lauder turned her bout with cancer into a formidable benefit for other women. I first met her when I was at an NIH conference on women's health in New York City. She is a striking woman and a proud survivor of the disease. No doubt influenced by her family's interest in cosmetics, she recognized the need for women to return to their regular activities as soon as possible, despite the insecurities many have about their appearance. Overcoming these insecurities is not always easy, and so Lauder set out to create a model of a comfortable environment with trained and supportive people to assist women in handling matters such as temporary hair loss or finding the proper prosthesis for a bathing suit. The Evelyn H. Lauder Breast Center at Memorial Sloan-Kettering, an integrated diagnostic and treatment center, offers women a wide range of services, including nutrition counseling, social services, psychiatry, and practical advice on adjusting to a changing body. This helps develop the confidence a woman needs to return to social and work life during therapy, and also in the longer term as a cancer veteran.

Jon Huntsman Sr. is another success story, turning his own good fortune in both health and business into the Huntsman Cancer Institute at the University of Utah in Salt Lake City. Huntsman lost both of his parents to cancer, and then went on himself to survive two life-threatening malignancies. As he has often said, "There is no one untouched by cancer—it respects no class, station, or age." His mission in building the Huntsman Institute was to bring cancer care with dignity to all patients, and to combine the cutting edge of research with a soothing place for cancer patients and their families.

It's no surprise that survivors from all walks of life, who are so keenly aware of what's at stake, have a yearning to help others, often in a spontaneous or anonymous way. Help might come from a next-door neighbor, a co-worker, or an unexpected visitor. I'm reminded of a friend my daughter Bartlett brought home for a visit one weekend. At one point we were gathered in the kitchen chatting away. I was in the midst of my chemotherapy but keeping that detail to myself. I had tucked away in the back of the refrigerator a vial of Neupogen, a medicine that builds up the white blood cells when your bone marrow is feeling blue. Only someone who knew how critical that drug could be—or what it represented—would have even noticed the obscure little vial. This young woman did. Here she was, the picture of good health, brimming with survivor savvy and telling me how she herself had become a master of her own self-injections with the drug years before, during a high school bout with Hodgkin's disease. She warmed my soul more than she ever imagined.

And who would have thought I would feel the same camaraderie with a woman I met only four months after becoming president of the American Red Cross, in the not-so-pleasant circumstances of a Food and Drug Administration inspection. The senior FDA investigator, a soft-spoken woman known among her peers as one of the most knowledgeable in the blood industry, recited the details of her scathing report to me and to several members of our top management and governing board. They included mislabeling, miscounting, and just plain missing units of blood and plasma; releases of tainted blood; and consistent failures to follow proper procedures for screening donors. These were problems, she firmly reminded the group, that had been identified in years past but still weren't being fixed. In her quiet, determined way she conveyed more than a scolding; it was worse. Yes, she was carrying out the duties of the federal agency she represented. But she was also deeply worried about the safety of individual donors and patients and was a staunch behind-the-scenes advocate for the millions of people who needed blood to survive, people who were trusting that it would be safe.

In the privacy of my office, the investigator told me that numerous blood transfusions had kept her alive during her own harrowing struggle with cancer—something she suspected I, too, had experienced. (Cancer patients are among the largest consumers of blood and blood products.) She had been a strong and tough inspector before that, but now she brought another dimension to her life's work. She reinforced to my team something that has been one of my teaching mantras for my entire career in medicine: if it's for the patient, always imagine you are that patient, and perform accordingly.

Survivor Groups on a Mission

This connection between survivors melts away position, age, gender, and ethnicity, and the passion that wells up has become the energy for the burgeoning number of community survivor groups. When Karen Jackson was diagnosed with breast cancer in 1994, it seemed to her that there was a dearth of resources available to black women such as herself. This wasn't really a subject that was being discussed openly in her community, and the support groups that did exist didn't seem like good options for her, either. On top of this, she was aware of the huge number of black women (and those who love them) who are affected by this disease. Jackson survived breast cancer and went on to found Sisters Network Inc., a national organization dedicated to educating African American women about breast cancer and offering support and empowerment to those who have been diagnosed with it. In a little over a decade, the organization has grown to include forty local chapters across the country. Jackson and her organization also initiated "Stop the Silence," a national campaign to reach out to black women in the 25- to 45-year-old age range who had no known history of breast cancer. Following in the path of Sisters Network, Thomas Farrington, a businessman from Boston and a prostate cancer survivor, started a brotherhood in 2003 called the Prostate Health Education Network to raise awareness of this disease among African American men and to provide support to survivors throughout the country.

This sort of can-do attitude is part of the American way; it personifies a history of social activism running through our culture. Certainly those in the breast cancer awareness movement took their cues from the AIDS activists of the 1980s and beyond, and borrowed some of those methods to get their message out to the general public. They in turn have inspired other advocacy groups. What begins with one person and a particular cause can mushroom into an entire movement.

The American Cancer Society's Relay for Life, one of its best-known events, began in May 1985 with a single person. Gordy Klatt, a surgeon and running enthusiast, spent twenty-four hours walking and running around a track in Tacoma, Washington, in order to raise money for that organization. Now these events can be found in 4,200 towns and communities across the country and in a number of foreign countries.

Patient activism of this type is in the genetic code of the American Cancer Society, an extraordinary and pioneering movement that early on marshaled the power of volunteerism. Founded in 1913 by a group of doctors and businessmen, the society, then known as the American Society for the Control of Cancer, was among the earliest of the community-based efforts to encourage the public to rally on behalf of a major health condition. Its symbol, which has endured since 1928, is a sword and a pair of serpents, very much heralding a nationwide public commitment to fight cancer as it would a war. According to the society, the sword represents the crusading spirit of the cancer movement and the two intertwined serpents of the medical caduceus that make up the sword's handle represent the healing of the sick and the creativity of the healthy—many of whom even back then (when such matters were not discussed) were survivors and members of their families.

Much of the society's success and its entrenchment in communities everywhere is credited to a group of women activists who in 1936 formed the Women's Field Army. The boldly named effort was the brainchild of Marjorie G. Illig, who worked with the society and chaired the General Federation of Women's Clubs Committee on Public Health. Her volunteers had one mission: to wage war on cancer. Accordingly, its recruits wore khaki uniforms dressed with insignias of their rank, and together they spearheaded a nationwide grassroots effort to educate the public about cancer and raise money for the society's work. These women in khakis not only turned the American Cancer Society into a major volunteer force but were the unheralded mothers of the war on cancer.

Many others have followed in their footsteps. More than twenty years ago, another survivor-advocate, Nancy Brinker, started the Susan G. Komen Breast Cancer Foundation in memory of her sister, who died of the disease. Brinker paid me a visit at NIH in 1992 on behalf of her foundation. Breast cancer had emerged from the shadows as a disease that women could talk about, and now efforts were turning toward spurring more research on the single most common cancer in women. Though she rarely focuses on it, Brinker herself is a survivor and has used the memory of her sister and her own personal experience and material resources to energize a broad-based, national foundation. Their efforts include running the National Toll-Free Breast Care Helpline, (800) IM AWARE, and overseeing various community-centered events around the country. The best known of these is the Race for the Cure, which occurs in over a hundred cities, involves more than a million people, and raises tens of millions of dollars each year to help fight breast cancer. Other organizations also sponsor walks or runs to raise money for cancer research and education; for example, the Avon Breast Cancer Crusade, sponsor of the Avon Walk for Breast Cancer, has given out over $400 million worldwide to fund breast cancer research and community health programs.

In addition to the Prostate Health Education Network, there are other prostate cancer survivors groups, including Man to Man (a program of the American Cancer Society) and Us TOO, which emulate the effectiveness of breast cancer activists in rallying for their cause. There are similar survivor-driven organizations for colon cancer (Colon Cancer Alliance) and thyroid cancer (ThyCa), and a survivor group is sponsored by the Leukemia and Lymphoma Society for blood cancers. But there are also organizations that focus on all survivors, regardless of their tumor type, including Gilda's Club, founded in the name of Gilda Radner, who died of ovarian cancer, and a nationwide organization called I Can Cope under the auspices of the American Cancer Society. And, of course, there's the Lance Armstrong Foundation; "Livestrong" may well be the best description for all of these many rallying efforts. It also has a survivor care program that offers advice on paying for treatment and other financial needs that arise.

There are many reasons why events sponsored by these various organizations are so popular. Aside from the obvious fund-raising aspect, these activities are a way for survivors to smile broadly and celebrate their health in solidarity with their loved ones. It's a time to

connect with other survivors, too. The experience can also be em-
powering, even to those who survey from afar the throngs of commit-
ted, vibrant people taking charge of their own health and channeling
their energy in a positive way to stand up to their disease.

A Longer View

Like any other large demographic, 10 million survivors makes for a
force to be reckoned with; the sheer numbers command attention.
On the medical care front, there has been a decided broadening of
focus from immediate treatment to a much longer view of cancer as
a chronic health issue. Now health professionals and most major
cancer centers are considering the complex medical, social, and psychological issues that arise when people live for years, even decades,
beyond their original cancer diagnosis. Programs for survivors uti-
lize a multidisciplinary approach, similar to that used in treating the
cancer in the first place.

Life after cancer has also made its way into the many reports of
government agencies such as the CDC and the NIH, charged with
tracking just where we stand as a nation in our battle against cancer.
Historically, these reports include a battery of statistics regarding
the number of new cases diagnosed and five-year survival figures, as
well as the number of deaths due to different cancers. The figures are
broken down by type of disease, gender, race—even state. Now
these reports are taking a longer view of the illness and examining
the long-term health outcomes and needs of survivors. For example,
a report of the President's Cancer Panel in 2004 called "Living
Beyond Cancer: Finding a New Balance" puts the spotlight specifically on survivors as a growing part of the war on cancer. With the
report's emphasis on the physical, psychological, and social issues of
cancer and its aftermath, this document addresses the needs and
concerns of all cancer survivors, regardless of where they are in their
cancer journey or what specific tumor brought them there.

A similar message is contained in "From Cancer Patient to

Cancer Survivor: Lost in Transition," released by the Institute of Medicine of the National Academy of Sciences. This 2005 report calls for greater awareness of cancer survivorship as a distinct phase of cancer care, a period that begins following first diagnosis and treatment and extends to cancer recurrence or death—and one that the Institute believes has been neglected. Part of the neglect, the report suggests, is a public queasiness with the word *survivor*, which is too closely associated with *victim*. Many people just don't want to carry that label. Europeans, for example, have been reluctant to use the term because cancer carries an even heavier social stigma there than it does in this country. For many patients here and abroad, the reason may be simpler and healthier than that: the determination many feel to just forget about a troubled time and move on.

However strong that impulse to move on may be, though, there are certain realities for all cancer veterans. Almost anyone who has survived cancer is at increased risk either of a recurrence or of developing another form of cancer. Whether that is due to family history or genetic predisposition, behavioral missteps such as smoking, or late effects of either chemotherapy or radiation on normal DNA is not the issue at this point. What matters is that a person once touched by cancer falls into a group that is at risk to be touched again. Consequently, he or she must adhere to cancer prevention strategies and be diligent about recommended follow-up cancer screening. Admittedly, there is always the deep-down angst that any visit to a doctor might turn up something. But the same general rule still applies: the sooner a malignancy is detected, the easier and more effective the treatment.

When I find myself covering up to walk on a sunny beach or fretting about a medical appointment a week before it happens, I remind myself that I am no different from a patient who has had a tussle with heart disease. If you've had a heart attack, you are at higher risk for flunking that next exercise stress test or for that minor twinge in the chest to be another coronary artery acting up, and those with coronary artery disease are more prone to strokes or aortic aneurysms. Thus most heart patients become wed to a program of ongoing prevention and medical surveillance. They know it is never too late to start, whether it's controlling their blood pressure or cholesterol, getting on the treadmill, or watching the waistline. The same is true for cancer, and the more we understand cancer as a chronic disease and develop treatment strategies to keep it in a state of enduring remission, the more the prevention mind-set will itself become enduring.

CHAPTER 15

Survivors All

SURVIVORS ARE EVERYWHERE, FROM your local shopkeeper to your child's teacher, your next-door neighbor to your own kitchen table. Among the most inspiring of them all are the children.

Childhood Survivors

Children who have taken the cancer journey are a special group as they ease back into their once-carefree lives. An obvious concern is how they manage the transition back to school and cope with making up for lost class time. They may have special needs arising from their illness or treatment, and they may experience developmental and/or social difficulties and require psychological counseling even after they've been pronounced cured. And, as always, their cancer affects the entire family.

Mixed in with their concern and fear, brothers and sisters may have complicated feelings about the "special treatment" the survivor has received. Siblings may resent, on some level, the attention their brother or sister is getting that may be detracting from their parents' ability to focus on the other children's needs. Parents, who have had to modify their own dreams and expectations, may require psychological support in order to cope with the difficulties of the child's illness along with all of the other demands on their time. Chronic illness in a child is often a source of marital strife, and negative feelings and resentments can linger long after the child is considered well. Parents and other family members need to come to terms with their own feelings before they can effectively help their children.

Let's not forget, though, that children are resilient; perhaps it's due to that blessed innocence they possess. Whatever the reason, they may be more adept at handling a cancer diagnosis than their parents are. One study of eight- to twelve-year-old cancer patients and survivors found that most were able to move on with their lives, without lingering psychological scars, once their treatments were over. By and large they were as content and well balanced as their peers who had never been ill.

Adolescents face their own challenges. This is a fragile time in children's development; they desperately want to fit in and be just like their friends. Receiving a cancer diagnosis and having to undergo treatment sets these young people apart, at least for a time. Because the peer group is so important at this age, friends can provide a level of comfort and support that parents sometimes can't offer. We see many examples of young people rallying around one of their friends or classmates who is facing cancer—a product of our willingness to talk more openly about cancer and to see the experience with more optimism than was the case even a decade ago. For example, we've heard of groups of young people who shave their heads in solidarity with friends who are undergoing chemotherapy treatments. In one Pennsylvania town, the school also got involved and used the head shaving as an innovative way to raise funds to defray the costs of an adolescent's medical treatment. While acts such as these can provide great comfort, they can't erase the fact that receiving a cancer diagnosis robs our children and young adults of a good hunk of their childhood. It forces them to grow up very fast. It's the goal of the medical community and of family and friends to ensure that the focus is always on a bright tomorrow, and on protecting that future each step of the way.

Invariably, cancer in the young comes as a bolt out of nowhere: perfectly innocent, healthy beings are struck by a potentially mortal illness at a time when mortality is not even in their vocabulary. What is so heartening is that some of the greatest strides have been made in the treatment of childhood and adolescent cancer. However, as many as two-thirds of young survivors have residual health issues that need to be addressed on a long-term basis, either due to these treatments or because of the cancer itself. Doctors are becoming increasingly alert to the physical and occasional psychological aftershocks, but parents need to be aware of them as well. Up front, families need to know about long-term side effects, including risks for second cancers, cosmetic issues that might need later attention, or concerns about the health of other organs in the body. All too often, reliable information is not readily available.

That's why the ongoing NIH-supported Childhood Cancer Survivor Study, begun in 1992 at the University of Minnesota, is so critical to the growing population of young veterans of cancer. The study has amassed over 20,000 patients gathered from twenty-seven cancer centers in the United States and Canada and compares them with a control group of 4,000 healthy siblings. The participants developed cancer at twenty years of age or younger, during the period 1970–1986, and survived more than five years after their cancer diagnosis. Along with detailed medical information, family history, and quality-of-life assessment, blood and tumor material have been banked for future biological and genetic analysis. This group of patients will be generously offering a vast treasure trove of information to guide pediatric oncologists, parents, and patients in delicately balancing the shorter-term benefits of cancer treatment with their longer-term effects. It is a gift from yesterday's cancer-stricken children to the children of tomorrow. And as more children and adolescents prevail over their acute illness, no doubt doctors will have the wherewithal to modify therapies appropriately.

But there is always a delicate balancing act when faced with a desperately ill child, and many of the later problems are the price of getting through the acute illness. Anyone who has dealt with young survivors has experienced the joy of bringing them enduring remissions and in some cases cures to otherwise fatal illnesses. Their parents see in their young troupers a heroism that they wonder if they could muster themselves. As these youngsters mature, they often show a sturdiness that comes from having overcome such a hurdle early in life. Integrating survivor health concerns into treatment plans is part of getting our young through their blackberry winter to grow strong and sturdy.

Adult Survivors

Cancer is still predominantly a disease of those over fifty years of age. For adults, dealing with a cancer diagnosis and the subsequent treatment and its follow-up may be just one more weight on already overburdened shoulders. And as more adults move past that five-year survival mark we're learning that their health needs, too, require a special kind of focus. Although not all survivors have to grapple with these aftershocks—and the majority I've encountered are grateful, if not exuberant, remembering the alternative—there may be residual problems that diminish with time, such as fatigue or low white blood cell counts. But there are also scars that don't go away, and a body that may not look like the one you expected to have.

Modern medicine offers many innovations to help survivors rehabilitate and return to a life of full living. Reconstructive breast surgery is a boon to many women after mastectomy, and drugs such as Viagra help survivors of prostate cancer deal with nerve injury that limits their sexual potency. Combating lymphedema, a congestion and often painful swelling of an arm or a leg—which can develop as late as four years after surgery or radiation treatments for cancer because of injury to regional lymph nodes and vessels of the lymphatic system—is a recognized component of rehabilitation services.

When cancer strikes a person of childbearing age, the ability to go on and have a family after treatment is an issue. If the cancer involves a woman's reproductive tract and calls for a hysterectomy, she is forced to deal with this loss from the outset, and her grief should not be underestimated or ignored. But for most survivors, having children after therapy is an option that is planned for with the help of sperm banking, ovary shields, and other advances in reproductive medicine. Nonetheless, impaired fertility or premature menopause can occur after certain chemotherapies, and most women who want to have children after treatment, with the counsel of their oncologists, are generally encouraged not to delay. Importantly, there is no evidence that children born to cancer survivors who have had either chemo or radiation are at risk for birth defects, or that women who become pregnant as cancer survivors face a greater risk of the cancer recurring.

A relatively new survivor issue is so-called chemo brain. For some survivors and some treatments, cognitive dysfunction can be an issue. Chemotherapy that blocks estrogen in the treatment of breast cancer, or testosterone as part of prostate cancer therapy, has been associated with memory problems or other subtle but noticeable declines in reasoning and organizational abilities. As mentioned earlier, brain radiation can inflame and sometimes permanently damage healthy brain tissue, leading to long-term cognitive decline, particularly when it involves large volumes of tissue. The reality is that we are still in the infancy of understanding neurodegenerative brain changes in general and how to alleviate or stabilize them, but patients and families need to be made aware of these potential effects of chemotherapy and radiation treatments.

Cancer survivors can encounter other health problems, including thinner bones, thyroid dysfunction, impaired breathing capacity, and heart failure. Again, these are risks of specific treatments, and even then not certainties, but such aftermaths call for ongoing medical attention.

For most people these added health risks are their quiet badges of courage. More than half of cancer survivors are over sixty, a time when everyone has seen some rough patches in life and probably lost a friend or loved one along the way. Their confrontation with disease and the recognition that they carry extra risks as a result is but another reminder that every day is a living day—and a precious one not to be squandered.

The Co-Survivors

While cancer survivors are a huge group, the estimate of 10 million does not include the full range of those touched deeply by the disease. Spouses and significant others, parents, and children can be caught up in the cancer trek, swept into a world that can transform their lives, too. The CDC, along with many individuals and organizations, such as the National Coalition for Cancer Survivorship, consider close relatives and friends to be survivors as well. The Komen Foundation calls them "co-survivors" and has a new initiative to offer them information and support. Similarly, the American Cancer Society's Cancer Survivor Network has online chat rooms, message boards, and Web pages celebrating the importance of these close relationships and offering inspiring stories of how people have been helped through their cancer trials with the care of loved ones. These people have provided a tender shoulder to lean on during a survivor's roughest ride; it's encouraging that their needs are being recognized, too.

The exhausted caregiver who is there lovingly through seemingly endless days and nights, the terrified child who watches in the shadows as a strong parent suddenly becomes weak, thin, bald, and unable to tend to the child's needs, and the parent whose angel-faced child is inexplicably taken ill—all have their own issues. They have lost their innocence, so to speak. Their lives are interrupted, their dreams put temporarily on hold. And they have gotten close to a nasty side of life that they hoped never to see. These memories linger.

My Genes, Your Genes

While we can control certain cancer risk factors up to a point, there's one we absolutely cannot control: our inherited genes. Co-survivors who are close relations are left with the inevitable question about their own vulnerability. There is already enough information out there about cancer genes for them to wonder what their own genes might have in store for them. And with this knowledge looms the issue of genetic testing.

A week does not go by when there is not another cancer gene identified that is shown to run in families. Over the past ten years, scientists have discovered a series of inherited genes for cancer of the breast, ovary, prostate, and colon. There are inherited genes that are linked to malignant melanoma and to rare tumors of childhood such as retinoblastoma, a cancer of the eye. The loss of the important tumor suppressor gene *p53* runs in families as a recessive gene (like blue eyes or blond hair) and creates a general state of increased cancer susceptibility. But as we have gotten smarter, we have learned that though these genes may bring increased risk, they are not the crystal balls we once thought. And that feeds into much of the ongoing debate about genetic testing.

The discovery of the *BRCA1* and *BRCA2* gene mutations is a case in point. The world cheered when scientists first isolated the *BRCA1* gene in 1994 and linked it to more than half of the cases of breast cancer that run in families. It was heralded as a great advance in medicine and made it seem as if a breakthrough in breast cancer treatment was imminent. One naysayer, Fran Visco, director of the National Breast Cancer Coalition advocacy group, seemed to be the skunk at that garden party. Yet her lack of exuberance had some basis. She asked plainly: What would this do for patients? Does it help? Are we closer to a cure? She was on to something.

Roughly 10 percent of the approximately 275,000 women diagnosed with breast cancer and the 22,000 women diagnosed with ovarian cancer this year can look to their genes as at least a co-conspirator. To be precise, these women (while there are some cases of male breast cancer, the disease overwhelmingly affects females) have inherited a gene from either their father or their mother that has been altered in such a way that the gene can no longer carry out its intended purpose: to hamper the development of cancer. But with deeper probing we find that there are 200 or more different mutations in the two *BRCA* cancer suppressor genes. There is no one culprit here. And as mentioned earlier, these mutated genes are not just about the breast. The variants may confer different risks for breast and ovarian cancer as well as for cancer of the prostate and colon—suggesting the *BRCA* name may have been given in haste. In addition, the same mutations in these genes can behave differently in different women. This is epigenetics at work, where factors or interactions not evident in the gene sequence itself influence how a gene expresses itself or otherwise behaves.

If anything, the early estimates linking the breast cancer genes to the development of breast cancer were overstated, and the isolated presence of such a gene itself says nothing. You still have to look at the complete picture of the patient and her family—and, ultimately and ideally, put it in the context of the entire genome for a given tumor type. The gene takes on meaning as a risk factor in a family in which several of its members have had breast or ovarian cancer; then the presence of the altered *BRCA1* or *BRCA2* gene marks a higher risk. This is also the case if the family has been cancer prone with other tumor types or is of Eastern European Jewish extraction. On the other hand, even if a person fits the above family profile and even if she (or he) gets cancer, it doesn't necessarily mean that she is carrying either of these genes.

So, what does the presence of one of these altered genes mean to the co-survivor kin? Yes, she faces a greater risk of developing breast or ovarian cancer in her thirties or forties; she may also have a greater risk of getting colon cancer, and male relatives with the *BRCA2* gene may be at greater risk for prostate cancer. But even then we cannot pinpoint the risk as precisely as once thought. Overall, a woman faces a lifetime risk of getting breast cancer of about 13 percent. If she carries the breast cancer gene, that risk rises, but with a broad range: anywhere between 36 and 85 percent. An even wider range exists for ovarian cancer, which according to the NCI has a lifetime risk of 1.7 percent in the general population. Here the estimates are that between 16 to 60 percent of women who carry the genetic change will be affected.

Now for the tough part: to test or not to test? Recognizing these widespread limitations, when does it make sense to look for inherited cancer genes, and how can the information be used? We certainly are not at the stage where random testing for a panel of cancer-related genes makes any sense at all. But for a family that is cancer prone, genetic knowledge can be helpful, since in the coin flip that comes with inheriting only half of either parent's genes, inheriting the cancer gene that may pepper any family's gene pool is no sure thing. The search for a cancer culprit gene should begin with the person who has had the cancer. If, for example, a woman with ovarian cancer is found to have an ovarian cancer–related gene, particularly in a family in which other close relatives have struggled with cancer, testing close family members can be of benefit. A positive finding in a sibling or offspring does not mean that a person will get cancer, but alerts him or her to an added *increased* risk and may be the extra stimulus needed to engage in earlier or more aggressive cancer screening—for example, PSA testing, colonoscopy starting before age fifty, or periodic pelvic ultrasound to examine the ovaries, which ordinarily is not a routine screening test.

But unless we can translate knowledge about inherited genes into a specific and positive action, getting this information for the sake of it, as I think Fran Visco was trying to point out, can have little value and may actually be destructive. Although some may feel better giving their offspring as much information as possible about what may lie ahead for them and their family's future generations, others may feel ambivalent about offering up this news. They may be haunted with the knowledge that they are a "carrier" of a disease-promoting gene and find it hard to live with the fact that they're at increased risk of getting cancer or of passing that risk on to their children. Assuming family members are already proactive about their health, even with this information there's not necessarily anything else that can be done to prevent cancer from striking. For anyone considering genetic testing, I would suggest that you think through what you will do with the results. The test itself is simple— one vial of blood—but the answers can be confusing. So if you proceed, do so under the guidance of a physician and a genetic counselor who will explore your entire family history and help you to interpret test results.

If the test for an abnormal gene is negative, meaning that the altered genes aren't present, that initial sigh of relief shouldn't obscure the fact that you still have a risk of getting cancer, although it's no different from that of the rest of the population. Getting a negative test result may make you think that you have escaped your familial risk (assuming others in your family have the gene), causing you to be less vigilant in your own cancer prevention and surveillance efforts. Also, there's a chance that you may be carrying a different mutated gene, for which you haven't been tested, that might increase your risk of getting cancer.

Another consideration that arises in this new world of gene discovery is whether or not one has an obligation to alert other close family members (siblings, children, parents) of a positive finding for a particular cancer-associated gene. That can be a family dilemma, however you play it. You may feel guilty for having passed on such a gene, but worse for being the messenger, having brought its presence in the family to light. Individual relatives may greet this news in varying ways, and you'll need to be prepared to deal with the fallout.

That's why drugstore kits for gene analysis, however likely they may be in our future, should not be seen as an advance to savor outside of the context of medical counseling and in full consideration of any action that might follow.

In some cases, those who have tested positive for a gene or gene profile associated with cancer opt for a prophylactic mastectomy or the removal of ovaries after childbearing. Those with familial polyposis bearing the APC gene are advised to undergo prophylactic colectomy (removal of the colon) after the age of forty. These surgical options seem drastic but ultimately come down to personal choice. The less onerous approach comes with preventive chemotherapy, as we've seen with tamoxifen for breast cancer, Celebrex for colon polyps, or vitamin C supplements for inveterate smokers at risk for lung cancer. These and many other agents will no doubt emerge as important adjuncts to reducing the risk of certain cancers, but current research is not conclusive on which patient groups will gain the greatest benefit, and their chronic use brings side effects of their own. There's also hope that down the road more targeted gene treatments will be devised using some of the novel small molecules discussed earlier in the book, such as RNA interference molecules. Or help may even come from a chemical found in your herb garden.

Aside from the personal and family issues raised by gene testing, there is also the ongoing concern about what happens if insurance companies, employers, or others become privy to this genetic information. It's possible that an insurance company might be influenced by the results of this test when deciding whether or not to offer life, health, or disability insurance; an employer might use this information to discriminate in some way. Although there are some laws already on the books regarding these issues, the laws aren't always so quick to match the advances in this evolving area of medicine. In general, when it comes to genetic testing, I would tread carefully.

Survivors' and Co-Survivors' Stake in Science

Regardless of how you feel about genetic testing, it's indisputable that unlocking the secrets of the multitude of cancers hidden in the genetic code is critical in our quest to conquer this disease. In the decades to come, this scientific exploration and the therapies drawn from it will increase exponentially. Science is the engine of progress. To bolster that belief, we need look no further than our own history as a country of discoverers and scientists; indeed, a passion for discovery seems to be a core American value.

But America's time-honored celebration of science has always had a practical bent. The patent system, embedded in Article I of our Constitution, is all about bringing scientific discoveries such as the cotton gin or the lightbulb to the public. President Franklin Roosevelt undoubtedly was thinking of defense research when he made the long drive from the White House out to the rolling hills of Bethesda, Maryland, to dedicate the campus of National Institutes of Health and the National Cancer Institute on October 31, 1940. Speaking from the portico of Building I (which is still the office of the NIH director), FDR pledged that our nation would devote itself to "life conservation, rather than life destruction." He knew about personal wars as well as world wars, suffering himself with high blood pressure, heart disease, and legs paralyzed by polio. In his glorious remarks, recorded for history and ones I've listened to more than once, he stresses a national need to apply science to both prevention and treatment of disease. He declared medical research to be a universal language of peace and humanitarianism, and that "we cannot be a strong nation unless we are a healthy nation."

These were no casual words at a dedication ceremony. Four years later, with our nation deeply embroiled in war, Roosevelt sent written instructions to his science advisor, Vannevar Bush, to develop a plan for civilian research after the war that would bring the power of science to domestic purposes, not just military ones. He called for a "war of science against disease," noting that deaths from one or two diseases, including cancer, vastly exceeded the numbers lost in battle. By that time Roosevelt was seriously ill with a failing heart and blood pressure out of control, which left him too weak to manage his heavy leg braces. Only months later he died of a stroke, four weeks before victory was declared in Europe. Roosevelt's NIH address and his letter to his science advisor did not get much attention at the time. But his plan was carried out by his science advisor and virtually all succeeding presidents.

Many other advocates kept this flame alive to form the medical research system we now enjoy. One of the earliest was the socially prominent philanthropist Mary Lasker, whose advertising executive husband, Albert, died of cancer. She became an outspoken patron of cancer research shortly after World War II and a benefactor of the American Cancer Society, who used her congressional contacts to gain support for what became an exponential growth in the NCI budget. The U.S. Congress, from both sides of the aisle, ensured an uninterrupted stream of support for medical research in this country. And it was with congressional commitment that President Richard Nixon officially declared the war on cancer in 1971, which set the National Cancer Institute apart from its peers in terms of planning, dollars, and White House oversight. Today, with an annual budget of $5 billion—rivaling the budgets of many small nations—the NCI is the focal point of the government's cancer research. Asked what his biggest accomplishments were as president, Nixon once replied to a former assistant that there were two: the opening of China and the war on cancer.

But with all these efforts going into cancer research for over half a century, there are many critics who believe the money has not returned what it should have by now. It's an understandable feeling for those who have not benefited from this war. However, the public has to know just how important their sentiments are to the pace of the fight; they are part of its energy, and such questioning is appropriate and constructive. Consider once more the Cancer Genome Atlas. Knowing the blueprints of different cancer genomes would offer a wealth of insight and new avenues for hypothesis building and drug discovery by the individual scientists in labs everywhere. We need to move more quickly with that effort.

Survivors and their families know urgency. They know cancer is a time bomb that is ticking not just for them but also for other people who just haven't figured that out yet. A perspective born of the very same common sense drove FDR to have faith that science would find something better, fueled by a passion that sprang from his own personal suffering. Many scientists are immersed in the cancer field because of its larger humanitarian goals, and they know the importance of moving quickly, but their own time pressures come mostly from peer competition—for recognition and money—that keeps the field of discovery dynamic. At base, though, the fire and sense of urgency that has made the NCI the largest of the NIH institutes come from a public singed by this illness one by one.

"If you build it they will come" is a formula that works in medical research efforts. We saw that happen when almost from nothing a multibillion-dollar research effort directed at HIV mushroomed in a matter of a few years. One cannot pursue expensive and important research, particularly in these times, unless there are substantial funds and a technical infrastructure to do so. And the public voice over the past half century has had enormous influence over the nation's investment in cancer research—more than most people may realize. If the cancer advocacy groups rally as one, they will make the decoding of cancer genomes happen sooner rather than later.

Informed cancer survivors, effectively communicating the power of science directed toward human health, are the best of all possible advocates for medical research. But the public has to be let in on the science, a long-established mission of the National Library of Medicine under the two-decade leadership of physician Don Lindberg. He dove into information technology before most even knew what the Internet was, giving the public and the medical community ready access to all published research through the library's PubMed system (www.pubmed.gov), discussed earlier.

The more one looks into the science of cancer, the more it becomes clear that it is just a matter of time before its secrets are found out. But time is the one thing survivors treasure above all else, and most know that their own remission may not last forever. The need for a renewed, fast-paced strategic assault on the tough cancers, the recurrent ones that do not always succumb to treatment the second or third time around, and on the disseminated ones is something in which every survivor—and co-survivor—has a clear and present stake.

Call to Arms: Peregrine's Way

Peregrine, the companion I found on my own journey, was first and foremost a cancer survivor, not a martyr. And he was a survivor on a mission—devoting his life to good works after his spontaneous remission. Perhaps one of his lessons is that all survivors, with their hard-won wisdom and insight, have the chance to offer up a few good works in whatever way they can on behalf of those who are struggling or will struggle with this disease. The cancer field has come as far as it has because of survivor and co-survivor energy— the energy of the Women's Field Army, the million Americans who flooded the Nixon White House with letters, and today the many millions of advocates who walk and run, write and speak out, fueling the fires of cancer research and its translation into patient good. With knowledge and communication at our fingertips, survivor power can be an even stronger force for change, focused on the universal goal of nothing less than figuring out how to turn around a cancer's aggressive march throughout the body. This is within our grasp. We must not be content to just hope for the day; rather, each of us must join the survivor crusade to see that it will happen—and in our lifetime.

PART SEVEN

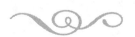

Attitudes of the Head and the Heart

Thence we came forth to rebehold the stars.

—*The Divine Comedy,*
Dante Alighieri

CHAPTER 16

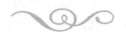

Weathering the Storm

HOWEVER PROMISING THE LATEST science, however smart and savvy the patient, cancer remains a journey of the heart and the spirit. For cancer takes you to a place that few diseases do. It forces you to confront your mortality, sometimes in a brutal and abrupt way, bringing into sharp focus just what matters to you most and what you might be losing. Cancer looms as something vague yet huge and terrifying, like an impending hurricane, still offshore but threatening to hit land soon. This emotional storm touches a common thread of humanity both in those who face the disease themselves and in those who witness and shiver at the thought that it might be lying in wait for them as well.

The fear and the dread of cancer run deep, obscuring the reality that today we are surrounded by millions of cancer survivors. Most will live for many years and, like Peregrine, fade away from other causes in ripe old age. Still, this fact brings limited solace, particularly early on in the cancer journey, because of the constant uncertainty each patient faces. It is always there, and confronting it can either bring fear or can inspire strength.

However severe the illness, our reactions to it are deeply personal— as personal as one's DNA. Yet the disease also forges a common bond that connects those who have walked its path. Not long ago, a colleague and I were talking about a mutual friend who was found to have a serious cancer; he looked at me and mused, "You know, those of us who have never peered across the River Styx are unable to fully understand what it is like to have done so. You are in a special and not so enviable club." On that score there is no better wisdom than that of the late Viktor Frankl, the renowned Viennese psychiatrist, philosopher, and Holocaust survivor who preached that everything can be taken away from a person except for one thing: the ability "to choose one's attitude in any given set of circumstances, to choose one's own way." He called this the "last of the human freedoms." The cancer patient always possesses this measure of control.

Confronting Fear

Choosing one's way and simply shutting the door on fear are not always easy to do. *Fear* is the word that pops up again and again as people talk about cancer. This fundamental emotion is often legitimate: fear of death, of disability, of unrelenting suffering and loss. The mind, however, does not adjust well to a chronic state of fear. Thus it is no wonder that many people put cancer talk out of their heads as much as possible—it's the mind's way of protecting itself from jarring thoughts. This may explain why some of the smartest people I know are unwilling even to schedule an appointment with their doctors, much less undergo cancer screening, or why some people almost by reflex keep their distance from those who are suffering with the disease. Cancer news can hit too close to home. Even television's Nielsen ratings demonstrate this fact, as I learned several years ago while working with CBS News as a medical consultant. My colleague Susan Zirinsky, the executive producer of 48 *Hours*, was planning to devote an entire show to cancer, as a public service. But she knew it was an iffy proposition because such programs usually bomb in the ratings. This struck me as odd, given that our nation's citizens so generously and faithfully support cancer research, more so than other diseases. What I learned is that confronting cancer in the abstract and at a distance is one thing. Facing it up close and personal, even on your TV screen, is quite another.

To be sure, news of cancer close to home is wrapped in sadness and anxiety, both for the patient and for the family. The news takes center stage as most other issues of the day melt away. In a millisecond all those affected are transported to a new and treacherous place. The world continues on, but the ones hearing the doctor's unhappy words suddenly feel like outsiders, with noses pressed up against a window, looking in enviously on a comfortable place that had once been theirs. They see a world churning about, caught up in shades of trivia, and wonder if they will ever be let back in. In this strange place, there seem to be no certain horizons. Call it alienation, disorientation, or just a sadness that wells up from knowing you are at risk of losing all that you have and love, all at once.

That sudden, stark imagining was something I had never encountered before receiving my own cancer news, yet in retrospect it was rather simple. Ordinarily when one experiences loss, it involves a single person or event. But to the individual facing such a stark time, whether sitting in a doctor's office, lying in a bed, or bleeding on a battlefield, the entire mortal world is threatened—family, friends, and all the everyday happenings of home or work. How could my children be without their chattering, pestering mom? And how could I do without my husband's guileless, wide-open grin that makes the sun come out? I was addicted to it, to the smell of his wonderful freshly ground coffee beans in the morning, and to the ever-changing look of his orchids, garden, and apple trees on our evening walks.

Fred insisted on those evening walks as therapy for my melting muscles. He would often ask me what I was thinking when, uncharacteristically, my idle chatter would fall quiet. But I never could tell him, back then, about the thoughts I had swirling around. Thoughts like, *If I'm gone, please don't move that painting of the two women and the baby from the bedroom wall even if you think it is a tad "womany."* Or *Won't you just hate opening day of football season without me?* Or *But of course you can toss out that dusty stack of journals in the corner of the family room that I cling to in my Irish housekeeping way.* I had already figured out that if I was going to be okay, these thoughts would have made me look like a drama queen. And if I wasn't, why would I let my gloom ruin a nice evening walk? While those closest to you may believe they understand what you're thinking, I'm not so sure they ever can. Like birth and death, this is one of the few life experiences you fundamentally face on your own; for, however many loved ones are around you, the cancer journey is essentially a solitary one. It's an existential experience in which past and future blend into the present moment. So much of who we are belongs to a future grown suddenly fuzzy. Losing control of that future, whatever the outcome, is disorienting to be sure, and can even be paralyzing.

Control What You Can

Treasuring the moment at hand and all that it contains for you is what lifts the spirit. Dismiss it as clichéd talk if you will, but to those threatened by a grave illness, every day of just being takes on a new light. Surely you wonder how you could ever complain again— about a rainy day, a broken piece of china, or someone's unkind words. Though that feeling of equanimity salves the cancer shock, it can also linger in the consciousness and become a subtle yet permanent state of being. I catch myself when I get too caught up in some silly little thing: I remind myself, *What am I doing? How lucky I am to be here!* One of my old friends, a long-term cancer survivor, and I find ourselves giving each other a knowing glance and an occasional high five to celebrate how fortunate we are, without needing to say more. That is the memory of a fear that has quieted, a terror that makes one fearless in the face of most other scares, a sadness that has taken its toll mildly, a dread that has enlightened mightily.

Your age and circumstance don't matter. Anne Marie Burns was just twenty-eight and a bride of three months when doctors gave her the shocking news that she had cancer—and not just any cancer, but a fast-growing tumor in her pelvis, one that would require immediate and unpleasant treatment. She was thrown into the scary and arcane world of cancer jargon: her tumor was unusual, saddled with the cumbersome name rhabdomyosarcoma. The standard treatment was the equally clumsy-sounding pelvic exenteration, the difficult reality I first encountered at the Boston Hospital for Women.

But her doctors at George Washington University Hospital in Washington, D.C., were aware that the childhood version of this cancer, which she appeared to have, responded well to nonsurgical treatment. Before proceeding, they formed a kind of brain trust, welcoming second opinions from two other major cancer centers, and even inviting Anne Marie's father, a physician, to be a part of their deliberations and decision making. After weighing her options, they decided to forgo surgery and treat medically, that is, with drugs and local radiation.

Talk about a stressful time for a young person! When I asked her how she managed the psychological burden, she told me, in her understated manner, that it was not the easiest way to spend the first year of marriage. But her husband was always supportive, she said, and they kept each other strong, never sinking too deeply into morbid thoughts. With insight rare for the young, she reminded me, "It was only a year, you know. We made the most of it, kept a positive attitude—and we laughed as much as we could."

Her family shared in both her faith and her good humor. Anne Marie relates how the Christmas after her October diagnosis, her mom stuffed her stocking with a little container of purple water labeled "Rhabdo Bug Juice." Later that Christmas Day, the whole family surprised Anne Marie by showing up at the dinner table wearing versions of the scarves and hats that she chose to wear during chemo, rather than the more conventional wig. Soon her friends began giving her odd hats and hatpins as gifts. Indeed, Anne Marie's offbeat headwear became her signature, her way of declaring, "Focus on the things that you can control." She now admits that she didn't really like the look, but "it was what I had to do."

Anne Marie says she tried hard not to feel sorry for herself, even though there were times she couldn't escape it. But her way was to be positive, and she made an active effort to keep the dark moments from taking hold. As she summed it up, "Cancer became my second job, but only my second job, since I realized that the treatment was temporary." She was right. Now, more than a decade later, she is cancer free. When others with cancer turn to her, she is always willing to share her experiences with them. Her advice? It's about funny hats, not tumors or treatment decisions. "Stay positive," she says. "Keep upbeat. Control what you can." When I suggested to her that she was a rather heroic young woman for keeping faith at such a time, she declined the compliment: "No. I had no other choice." As for fear, she did not allow herself even to think about it.

Life plays out in strange ways, and so it has been with the intertwining of Anne Marie's cancer story and my own. When I got the bad news of my illness that Valentine's Day many years ago, kind and gentle Dr. Sweeney also told me about his young daughter—and that she was now thriving despite the shocking discovery of her rare, life-threatening cancer. It was Anne Marie. She did not know the comfort she brought me that dark night. Much later, I asked her dad if I could speak with her directly. Then I was finally able to say thank you: for her dad, but also for her strength and wisdom, which warmed my heart.

I find myself returning to Anne Marie's story because it contains a nugget of universal cancer wisdom that is inescapable and worth repeating: be constructive and grasp the positive in whatever you hear. I know some studies claim that a positive attitude has no bearing on the outcome of one's illness, but I don't entirely buy that. I believe that it is a key determinant of your quality of life following diagnosis. And that there is no reason to assume the worst outcome any more than there is to blindly assume the best. Some patients complain that they do not want to pretend to be positive when they really feel so down and rotten. Or, worse, they become guilty about their negativity and fear that it will cause them further harm. Fair enough, but remember that dread and sadness are not sustainable states of being. And one does not have to be a blind Pollyanna to think *living time* and make a conscious decision to value every moment of it. As Anne Marie puts it, "Even when I go back for regular checkups, I'm confident—but never overconfident." What it means is that you have learned what most people ignore: that when you feel life's mortality in the marrow of your bones, you value life all the more. It is not constructive to squander something so valuable by wallowing in the darkness of despair.

We each find ways to handle these hard times. One of my coping mechanisms is a simple mantra: "showtime." It comes with a history. "Showtime" is the name of a little bronze statue of a clown that my husband and I found in a small gallery in New York more than twenty years ago. After we brought the piece home, I called Peggy Mach, a little-known artist at the time, wanting to learn more about her magical and mysterious little beauty. The clown has a smooth cap with a graceful widow's peak and cheeks painted with red hearts. With a delicate turn of her wrist, she's using a long paintbrush to put lipstick on her softly smiling mouth as she gazes into a bronze mirror. In the mirror you catch her eyes, and they startle with their sadness. The artist told me the little clown emerged after an *annus horribilis* during which her husband had some personal difficulties and she had suffered paralyzing artist's block. One day she went into her studio and from the clay emerged the pretty little clown, smiling with mournful eyes. She called the work "Showtime." Whatever is afoot, whatever is lurking down deep, put on your lipstick and smile for those around you. So many times during my own *annus horribilis* I whispered to myself, "Showtime."

It was not always easy to follow this mantra, but somehow it worked. And it was reminiscent of one of my own pearls of wisdom that I used to teach students and residents as we made the rounds of the cardiac care unit back in my Johns Hopkins days. I called it the positive lipstick sign (for women, of course). In the morning, if your patient is sitting up in bed with her lipstick on, you can be sure that she is feeling better—even before you examine her, and even if her eyes are a little sad.

～ FINDING YOUR WAY ～

Cancer's path can be rocky, and each of us needs to find our own way in what is an intensely personal experience. I found it helpful to think through just how I would try to help a patient face what I was facing.

~ *Catch your breath.* Your mind is racing and needs to take a pause. Ask a lot of questions, talk things over with your loved ones, and don't make any snap decisions. There's almost always time to mull things over, and get another opinion if you wish to. And if you can, try not to let your illness become more than your second, part-time job.

~ *Control what you can.* A cancer diagnosis is a setup for feeling helpless. Someone else and something else has taken over your body, and while those around you all seem so strong, you feel so weak. One very smart patient told me how he hated suddenly being treated like a child. If that's on your mind, have a frank discussion with your family and your health care team about it. Decide what it is that you can or want to weigh in on about your medical journey and your personal life. That includes what you want to tell others about your personal health: whether to discuss it or keep it private should be under your control, too. The goal is to wear your own hat, not someone else's.

~ *Stay constructive.* It's not easy to think constructively when you're facing something that seems so destructive. Whatever the circumstances, keep reminding yourself that how you react will influence how others react to you, and both will influence how you feel and live. As a matter of policy, assume that you will do at least as well as the best of those who have had your disease before, not as badly as the worst. Remember most of all that every day is living time.

~ *Avoid the anger trap.* We are all human, and it is easy for fear and anxiety to morph into anger, depression, and grief over what is being threatened or taken away. But cancer diagnosis can trap patients on an emotional roller coaster, with negative feelings spiraling into their own reality. Try and remember that the fury of "Why me?" is answered just by looking around at the many afflicted with devastating illnesses or other random misfortunes. The more apt question is: "Why not me? Why should I be spared?" Cancer specialists understand the cancer fury, and support groups, counseling, or medication can help. Your feelings are predictable, not shameful—but it's important to control them.

~ *Look for the humor.* If you have even a little funny bone, now's the time to use it. There is nothing funny about cancer, but because of it you may find yourself in some pretty silly situations—if only you can laugh at yourself and the world around you. You have earned the right to be deliciously irreverent. This will also help you to cope with those who sometimes fumble in trying to deal with your illness.

~ *Insist on respect.* Perhaps it's obvious, but you need a health care environment that does more than treat your body. Most health professionals have chosen medicine because of their profound respect for human dignity and their desire to help the sick. But if you find yourself in an environment that does not meet your emotional needs, find one that does. Even if it's at an institution or with doctors that have been touted as the best, keep in mind that there are many "bests" in today's medical world.

~ *Nourish your spirit.* Religious faith or spirituality often wells up in troubled times, and some studies claim that it is the most common if not most successful complementary medicine we have going. Even among those who are proclaimed atheists, when faced with cancer, dormant spiritual feelings or beliefs sometimes emerge. This is not something that you can or should force, but don't underestimate or undervalue its power to bring solace or balance when it is there.

Dealing with the So-called Stigma

Perhaps the hardest part of maintaining the right attitude is finding polite ways to deal with the silliness of others. People with cancer cannot fall prey to others' cancer phobias, which can stigmatize; the myths, which can confuse; or poor etiquette, which can drag you down. Sometimes people are literally afraid to extend a hand to others with cancer, as if they were lepers. Though intellectually we all know that cancer isn't catching (with the exception of the handful of infectious diseases that increase the risk for certain cancers, as noted in Chapter 6), historically it has been one of those illnesses that repels people. As Susan Sontag wrote in her classic book *Illness as Metaphor*, the disease was "felt to be obscene—in the original meaning of that word: ill-omened, abominable, repugnant to the senses." The treatments were rough on the body (though they are less so now) and often permanently disfiguring. For the longest time, cancer wasn't openly discussed, perhaps because, as with mental illness, people felt too ashamed to talk about it. That silence came at quite a cost: not only did it prevent the public from becoming educated about the disease, it also denied people the chance to offer support to those suffering from it, adding further to the burden of the ill.

Those days are blessedly over, by and large, thanks in part to First Lady Betty Ford, who in 1974 disclosed the fact that she had breast cancer. This brave admission jump-started a national conversation, helping people everywhere to understand the actual facts about the disease, and paving the way for the work of various organizations whose public service campaigns provided an education about the warning signs of cancer. In her strong but quiet way, she— and her daughter, Susan Ford Bales, who has picked up the torch— has saved countless lives and brought solace to many.

People with cancer no longer hide out during treatments, shy away from social events, or rush to quit their jobs as soon as they are diagnosed. In fact, more people than ever are able to continue working while they're undergoing treatment. In general, the workplace offers a friendlier, more sympathetic environment than it used to. Most employers offer flex time and other arrangements for those juggling treatment schedules and work and family responsibilities. Often employers have no choice in the matter because some of these workplace accommodations are now mandated by state and federal laws.

But a certain stigma lingers. An oncologist friend of mine who had her own bout with cancer confided to me shortly after I fell ill that she never told any of her colleagues about her diagnosis for fear that it would harm her professionally. She was certain that even in her field, working with other medical experts who should know better, she would be marginalized. She might not be offered the same professional opportunities as others. The focus would be on her breasts, not on what she'd accomplished and what she could accomplish. It was not that her position wasn't secure; she was a tenured professor. Rather, she worried she'd be placed in a lesser category of being, a category defined by her illness.

Were her fears justified? It's hard to say. Many cancer patients worry that they bear a big scarlet C on their chests, a virtual mark that makes them feel vulnerable to discrimination. But unlike poor Hester Prynne in *The Scarlet Letter*, the stigma is not always imposed by others. At least some of it comes from within and calls for an internal attitude adjustment, too. Early on in my cancer journey, I couldn't shake the feeling that I had somehow let people down. I felt so bad for my husband, who'd had the misfortune to marry someone like me. We'd always been equal partners in the relationship, and I'd always pulled my weight, but now I was going to be the proverbial albatross around his neck. I wondered if he would have married me had he known I was destined to have this terrible cancer. And then there were my children. I was letting them down, too, and that was pure agony. Would they regret having me as their mother? Clearly, I was at an especially vulnerable point. Though I know now that they felt no such thing, back then I often found myself doing something silly just to prove my value.

I went so far as trying to be handy, a new role for me. I've never been Ms. Fix-it. In fact, my mechanical ineptness is a longtime source of family amusement. There was this one recalcitrant drawer that just wouldn't move freely. Fred tried, my girls tried, but no one could get it to work properly. For some reason I became determined to fix that blasted drawer. Within hours of returning from a brief hospital visit to have some chemo-related blood work done, I found myself down on the floor, surrounded by tools, pulling and prying and reassembling odd little metal bits, until I managed to fix the darn thing and get it gliding smoothly on its rollers. When that drawer opened I felt a surge of joy: I was still a functioning part of this family, and here was physical proof of that. In retrospect, I understand that that silly drawer underscored how low my self-esteem had fallen. I had bought into the cancer stigma, at least for a little while.

Cancer Myths

Like all illnesses, cancer comes with its own set of myths. In retrospect, I realize that I was guided by my own myth—the doctor's myth, perhaps—that as long as I followed my own good advice I would be spared this disease. So I'm not surprised that studies have turned up a lot of misinformation about cancer in the minds of the public. Some myths are harmless, but others can disillusion or lead cancer patients down the wrong treatment path and are worth correcting.

According to a recent survey by the American Cancer Society, 41 percent of those queried believed erroneously that surgery can cause cancer to spread. More than 10 percent thought that the only thing needed to beat cancer was a positive attitude. And perhaps most startling, one in four thought the medical community actually had a cure for cancer in hand but for financial reasons was withholding it from the public. Other myths include the mistaken belief that individuals with certain types of personalities, such as those who are self-sacrificing caretakers or passive and repressed, are more likely to get hit by cancer (see Chapter 6). Or that visualizing the "good" cells gobbling up the bad—however soothing a thought that was to me—will help those good cells along. Some people believe that alternative medicines are of equal value to the conventional medicines, even if there have been no research studies to back this up. I guess some of these ideas are no less far-fetched than the ancient theory of the bodily humors, taken as medical gospel for centuries but now totally discredited. Would that cures were as easy as dredging black bile from your system.

Another notion that refuses to die—and needs to—is that people somehow cause their own cancers. I know people who can't shake the feeling that they are sick because of negative emotions, or drown in self-blame for the cancer risks they flirted with in the past. Even if unhealthy behavior has contributed in some way to one's illness, that does not mean it is the sure cause. Most with the same bad habits still dodge the bullet. Despite this fact, when we hear that someone has lung cancer, invariably the first question asked is "Does he or she smoke?" as if inhaling would explain away the illness and therefore justify a tempered sympathy. Sure, smoking increases your chances of getting many cancers, but for those with cancer it isn't terribly productive to be awash in guilt and self-recrimination. Remember, about 30 percent of those with lung cancer have never smoked, yet even they all too often find a less-than-sympathetic world when their cancer appears in the lung.

Our blame-game culture informs our perspective on many other threatening diseases as well, including heart attacks and other illnesses in which there are identifiable health risk factors. Just recently I lost my sister Michele, a quiet free spirit who brought a lot of joy to our world. When I spoke to a distant relative who had not seen her in over a decade, her first comment was "I'm not surprised. She never took care of herself." Boy, is that an overused line, perhaps betraying the blamer's hope that it couldn't happen to her since she does it right. If only we mortals had such control over our destinies. In fact, we all have our share of vices, but, as discussed, aging is the biggest risk factor of all for getting cancer. When faced with a fallen friend or loved one, patient or distant acquaintance, it's far better to channel one's energies in a more constructive and compassionate direction.

Cancer Is Not a Win-or-Lose War

Have you beaten it? Are you cured? The cancer-as-war metaphor paints the disease as an enemy that must be totally vanquished. You win or you lose. You're cured or you're doomed.

But one of the main benefits of understanding cancer on a molecular level is to recognize that cancer's secrets are to be found in all of our self-replicating and sometimes fragile DNA. Some cancers come and go without our knowing. Others can be watched cautiously because they are slow-growing and unlikely to bring trouble in one's natural life span.

When viewed from this perspective, it becomes clear that while we may not be able to defeat cancer, we can tame it and keep it in check. And control can be as good as a cure when therapies bring longer and longer remissions. Where the goals in cancer's war were once limited to preventing and eliminating the disease, now they have shifted to include the biological or chemical control of cancerous cells that cannot be entirely eliminated. A manageable, chronic condition is a victory in the new lexicon. Surely the idea of living well with cancer brings its own psychological implications and calls for a fundamental recalibration of attitude.

Cancer Etiquette

There is also a certain black humor in this journey. No doubt every cancer survivor has his or her own list of unforgettable exchanges with friends and associates, the dumb things people say with the best of intentions. How about this welcome greeting to one patient who had just learned of a serious cancer: "My, you don't look so bad." And a kind note of solace: "I hope you don't suffer too much." A concerned query: "Does it hurt?" Or the ever popular "Is that your hair?"

Then there was the night my husband and I had to attend an out-of-town work-related black-tie affair. I was in the midst of my second cycle of chemo. I'd lost a good deal of weight but wasn't feeling too bad. I managed to pull myself together and don an appropriate outfit, along with makeup, jewelry, my fanciest shoes, and a heavy dose of hair spray to obscure my thinning mop. As we were leaving the hotel, I caught a glimpse of us in the hall mirror. *Okay,* I thought, *I can do this.* There were nearly a thousand people at this event. Usually Fred is the one who wants to leave this sort of affair first, but I could barely endure the cocktails, endless courses, and many speeches. I would periodically lean over and plead with him, as our kids would when they were little: "Can we leave now?" Wiser than I, he encouraged me to hang in until it was not too obvious if we left.

Nonetheless, we were among the first to bolt. We ran into a colleague and his wife, also early escapees, and we all piled into one of the waiting cars. No sooner had we taken off than my colleague's wife, whom I barely knew, began to babble exuberantly, leaving me to respond only in my mind. First she said brightly, in a complimentary tone, "You look great. It's amazing how good you can look when you're dying!" (*Gee, thanks,* I thought.) In the next breath she told me that her mother had died a few years ago, and that her father had remarried within six months of her death. "Don't you think that was a sign of how much he loved my mother?" (*Sorry, don't agree,* I thought as I glanced over at my husband, looking especially handsome in his tuxedo, engaged in his own conversation about something more apropos, like the weather.) Her next words of wisdom: "But we all die sooner or later, don't we?" (*You betcha; heard that before.*) By the time we got to the hotel it was sinking in how funny the whole interchange had been, and I couldn't wait until we got to our room so I could tell Fred of my la-la land encounter. He laughed, too, but reminded me sweetly that the poor lady meant well.

After a while you get used to such comments—though not entirely. Not long ago, an old colleague of mine, whom I had not spoken to in a while, ended our phone conversation on another topic with an out-of-the-blue "How *are* you? Everyone else wants to know but is afraid to ask." Curiously, cancer seems to be a magnet for this kind of bizarre etiquette. You don't hear it if you've got a broken hip or survived a heart attack or even a heart transplant. I have concluded that it stems largely from that instinctive fear that a cancer diagnosis equals death, inspiring a kind of psychological rubbernecking. It's a primal emotion, no doubt, but one that needs to go the way of the dodo bird. When it comes to cancer, we are in a different era. Of course, as my husband pointed out, the klutzy remarks are well intended, and I suspect they are a reflection of the person's own insecurity and anxiety. Buried in there, too, may be a trace of that inevitable "Better you than me."

Whenever I hear one of these well-intended but insensitive remarks, I remind myself that living long is the best revenge. And until the etiquette mavens weigh in with their expertise, let me offer some basic advice we'd all do well to remember. If you want to reach out to someone who is facing cancer:

~ Do speak from the heart. A few tender sentences (either spoken or written) will resonate long after the many well-intentioned platitudes have been forgotten. How about "You're the best" if it's true, or "You can count on me" if you're sure.
~ Do think before you speak or write that note. You may think you're being kind, but are you? Your friend is dealing with a serious illness, but it hasn't transformed her into an infant, an imbe-

cile, or a corpse. Try something like "I can only imagine how tough this is, but I respect how you have faced this time and admire your strength. Love to you and your family," provided, again, that it's true.

~ Don't be afraid to praise the heroism of the person facing cancer. It can be a hellish road, and there's no need to tap-dance around this fact. When I became ill, one of our good friends, Mal Mixon, sent me a handwritten note. He tenderly reminded me of his own recovery after a grim battle with testicular cancer some thirty years before. Nothing patronizing, no pity, just a gentle encouragement: "I know your strength; you can do it, too, Bernie."

~ And please, don't be too quick to write off your fallen comrade or to try and calibrate how many months he has left on the planet. The answer is *always* that we do not know. Cancer has a mind of its own. In this context, banish the following from your vocabulary: *terminal*, *incurable*, *hopeless*, and *salvage*. How you think and talk will influence how you relate.

Perhaps the best piece of advice I can give is to imagine, as best you can, that you are the patient. Make sure that what you're offering will enhance the person's sense of well-being. This happens when what you say instills hope and faith. You don't discourage a person from running a marathon by saying, "It's too hard," "You haven't trained enough," or "Why on earth would you want to do that?" Instead, you encourage along the lines of "We're rooting for you," "I admire your determination," or "We know you can do it." If you're still not sure that what you're about to say will be received in the way it's intended, then don't say it. A simple hug or a "thinking of you, dear friend" note can mean a lot, too.

CHAPTER 17

Living Time

FOR A WHILE, LIFE to me seemed to fall into two time zones: B.C. was the time before my cancer diagnosis; A.C., the time after. I quickly learned that this sensibility was not just mine alone, as my illness touched everyone in the family to a greater or lesser extent.

When I fell ill, my sister Michele came right over in the middle of the night to be with our ninety-eight-year-old Nonie, who was soundly sleeping, and our twelve-year-old Marie, who was wide awake and terrified by the frightening sight of her mom being carried off in an ambulance. The next morning, after returning from the hospital, my husband sat with Marie at the kitchen table and calmly told her about the tumor. He said that I was doing fine but would have some difficult times ahead. What she remembers most about that conversation was her dad saying, "Marie, today is the day you grow up."

I've asked her if that was burdensome. No, she said. Instead, she felt that this was the first time Dad was confiding in her like an adult. But she quickly added, with her inviting, devilish smile, that it didn't take long to snap back into her soon-to-be-teen ways the moment she saw me going about my business and looking okay.

Our older daughter, Bartlett, came right home from college to be with me during the time of the operation. She, too, had to swallow some hard truths and assume a degree of responsibility well beyond her years. Not only did she comfort Marie when she couldn't sleep, but she gave me one of the most beautiful gifts I have ever received. It was that exquisite letter I mentioned in Chapter 2, which I continue to cherish to this day. In her handwritten note she acknowledged how hard it was for her to accept my diagnosis, and that this was a time when I, too, might need a shoulder to lean on, and offered me hers. And then she promised me the one thing she knew would mean the most to me: if something happened to me, she would not only look after her younger sister but support her in the strong, compassionate, and loving way that I had tended to her. Our children still in the nest, or even those just starting to fly away, suffer in their own ways when they are hit with sudden vulnerability in their parents. In their world, Mom and Dad are the supports they should just take for granted; it's traumatic to have that threatened. There is an old Jewish proverb that speaks to this: "When the father looks after the son, both smile. When the son looks after the father, both cry."

Parents of adults with cancer have their own burdens. It is not supposed to be that parents outlive their children, and both my mother and mother-in-law, who were part of our extended nest, suffered through my illness sometimes more than I did. I was disrupting the normal order of things. Michele would quietly tell me of the struggles that they tried so hard to shield from me; and I could see that Mom, Michele, and Nonie were my hovering guardian angels. However you look at it, cancer touches the psyche of the whole family. That can make for a strangely beautiful and family-affirming time.

To be sure, every family is different in the way it handles intense stress and uncertainty; it depends in part on the nature of the preexisting relationships, on temperament, and maybe even on gender. The way my husband, Fred, dealt with the news of my illness was never to lose faith that I'd be fine, and to keep me from wandering into the dreary world of what-ifs. He was my protector-in-chief but never made me feel like an invalid or less of a person because of my illness. And he never ceased to talk about tomorrow. Though there were times when I wanted to say, "But I'm not fine, can't you see?" to him I was always just fine, and that helped me as I tried to keep it that way.

A few years after my recovery, we were at a professional event where we were socializing with a British colleague of Fred's. His wife, in the midst of treatment for ovarian cancer, was not with him. Perhaps because he knew that we had gone through this, too, he told us about her illness and his optimism about her progress so far. He confided, rather tenderly and with a look of uncharacteristic puzzlement on his face, that his wife told him he didn't understand what she was going through. Fred looked at him sympathetically, then at me, and remarked with a little chuckle, "They all say that!" What I could see in these sweet men were two successful, protective, take-charge surgeons who wished to dwell only on the positive, on the concrete, on solving the problem, and on what could be controlled—not on dreary uncertainties.

I am, however, the first to recognize that talking through what might be—both the good and the not-so-good scenarios—and taking on cancer as a joint effort works wonders for many people. Penny and Bill George will tell you that working through her experience with cancer changed both of their lives. Penny, a psychologist by training, was convinced she would die when she first faced an early but invasive breast cancer. But her husband, Bill, CEO of a major medical technology company, refused to go to that gloomy place with her. "I missed that he was as frightened as I was. He was traumatized but did not show it," Penny said. At first, that is. Now it seems that her cancer journey became a mental and spiritual transformation for them both. When complementary medicine was just beginning to come out of the closet, Penny, with Bill's encouragement, embraced—along with conventional treatments—many forms of alternative healing: meditation, massage, acupuncture, experimenting with natural herbs for symptom control, and a deeper level of spirituality. In her quest to put meaning into this time in her life, she realized, "I felt no passion in my psychology work. I had to do something different." She relates that Bill and she began to think a lot about whole-person healing, and that led them to a richer and more purposeful way of living. How so? "Less automatic behavior, and focusing on what we believe is nourishing and what is intentional rather than what is only reactive or what you feel obliged to do because someone else is asking."

Penny goes so far as to say, "Cancer was the best thing that happened to me" and "Yes, I thought about dying and I'm glad I did." Now, more than ten years after the discovery of her cancer, she describes herself as more self-confident and less fearful because of it. Understanding and teaching about what she describes as a transformative experience is her new passion. The Georges devote both labor and financial support to the Bravewell Collaborative, a group of philanthropists Penny was instrumental in pulling together, with the mission of advancing integrative medicine for both wellness and healing. As I have watched their journey over the years, I've often thought that Penny and Bill's team approach was not unlike couples taking Lamaze classes together. They coach each other in the affirmative and life-enhancing ways that enable them to face pain at a time of birth—or rebirth.

But these are also the times that can make people fall apart or fall away from each other. Most physicians who deal with the seriously ill know of the many complex family dynamics—both good and bad—that can emerge. I concluded long ago that heart attacks either bring families together or tear their hearts apart. It's the same with cancer, only more so. Emotions churn, futures become uncertain, day-to-day routines are upset, and sometimes financial problems rear their heads. This can easily be a formula for creating distance, not closeness; for avoidance, not intimacy. The healthy want to get on with their lives—or is it that they are frightened themselves and have trouble coping with their own emotions while they are expected to be supportive of another?

As Harvard oncologist Jerome Groopman sees it, cancer's occurrence in a family member or close friend "holds up a mirror, a mirror of their own vulnerability. Some recoil from that mirror." He has seen the destructive effects of cancer stress on families and relationships more than once. Sometimes there are problems in the relationships to start with; sometimes it's the underlying nature of one or the other person that they just cannot take on the burden of illness, whatever was said in their vows. I asked him about the young woman he wrote about several years ago in one of his essays in the *New Yorker*. She was found to have advanced breast cancer that shortly took her life, but in the midst of it all she was abandoned by her fiancé. Good riddance, of course, and fortunately her family was there to catch her. In that instance, Groopman said the fiancé was a selfish and shallow character who bolted at the first hint of adversity. Everything in his life had been picture perfect; then suddenly it was not. Her illness uncovered a fragile relationship that broke apart during a difficult and trying time. As Groopman points out, in some cases the abandonment can be emotional, not physical. He recalls one terribly obnoxious, hard-driving venture capitalist whose metastatic cancer only made him more demanding and difficult, including toward his wife, whom he treated like a doormat. His kids wouldn't visit him, but she would dutifully come to his treatments and sit there coolly and silently knitting—like Madame Defarge in Charles Dickens's *A Tale of Two Cities*.

Fortunately, most of the time, families manage through the stress of illness. It's hard for doctors to step in even if they see the family train wreck happening. But most cancer centers have special family counseling programs and other social services that can provide emotional support to families and help family members understand what's happening before relationships come unglued. Support groups and mentors, as discussed earlier, can also help ameliorate what is still a strained situation and not yet a broken one. I'd also vote for some preventive medicine. Though one never knows how he or she will react under fire, there is good reason for couples and families to periodically take a deep breath and ponder in health just what that vow "in sickness" really means to them. Tipping my hat to the opening sentence of Tolstoy's *Anna Karenina*, there are two kinds of families: the ones that pull together with a remarkably similar focus on hope and love when one of their members is ill, and those that, instead, fall apart in all sorts of different and painful ways. It's good to know where you stand.

On Living and Dying

Fred and I have known Ray Klimczuk for many years. He lost his wife, Marge, to ovarian cancer when she was fifty-four. With enduring admiration he speaks of her courage and calmness during that time, and believes that her secret was that she never got off the "reality bus." In fact, as he puts it, she led the parade. She shaved her head before she lost her hair. And she wrote thirty-five letters to loved ones and friends in the weeks before she died, for her husband to distribute after her passing. In big, easy, undisturbed penmanship, she wrote messages of thanks, expressing not grief but gratitude. And she prayed a lot, too. Of all things, St. Peregrine was one of her favorites. Ray knew that St. Peregrine had a remission from his cancer, and he is quick to point out that "Marge and I had a year of remission." To him their time together back then was worth an eternity. Marge died at home with her family around her, drifting in and out of consciousness, holding Ray's hand, telling little jokes, and uttering in a final whisper, "Hi, Mom!" She left her family with the comfort that she had gone over to see the mother she'd lost to lung disease when she was a young woman.

Immortality is not an option for any of us, and there comes a time when even the best treatments of the day fail, when all reprieves are exhausted. Anyone who faces cancer knows for real that it is always lurking in the shadows, and a career in medicine teaches you that life deals rough hands to everyone sooner or later. But I'll say it again: you can choose how you deal with a bad hand even in the face of death. On that score I have seen many courageous and inspiring patients who are able to expect the best, treasure what they have, and deal with the unexpected as it comes. That is as good a formula as I know.

Back in the 1960s, Elisabeth Kübler-Ross defined the emotions of dying based on her own research in psychiatry. A Swiss-born psychiatrist working at the University of Chicago, Kübler-Ross is perhaps best known for her book *On Death and Dying*, which identified five stages patients go through when facing death: denial, anger, bargaining, depression, and acceptance. With this systematic focus, she taught us that the dying process needed to be part of medical care—part of healing. Her work informs a field of psychology known as thanatology, after the Greek god Thanatos, who in ancient mythology brought death to mortals.

I was first introduced to the relatively new field of thanatology when I was in medical training, and I have to confess that its name still gives me the creeps. Back then I also struggled with the notion that stages of death and dying were the same for all patients, regardless of their circumstance or illness, for even during my early student encounters with the critically ill, I saw a much broader range of emotions pouring out of human hearts that didn't always fit the rigid formula. My views have not changed much since then. While I don't doubt that people have many of these feelings and sometimes even in the prescribed sequence, in my experience patients die in much the same way as they have lived: as complex and wondrous individuals with a wide array of responses to misfortune.

Perhaps the five-stage psychological formula, when interpreted too literally and without nuances and texture, is a vestige of yester-day's response to cancer treatment, which tries to cram everyone into the same box. If interpreted too rigidly, it puts yet another bur-den on a person who has received a cancer diagnosis, stifling a sense of hope and the possibility for recovery. For some, this psychologi-cal formula may seem fatalistic and discouraging as they try to live as rich a life as they can for however long that may be. Is there ever a time when the human soul should abandon hope? To me, not even at the moment of that final breath.

But let's consider Kübler-Ross's five stages as they might apply to cancer in today's light.

~ DENIAL. When you're first told that you have a potentially fatal disease, it's probably natural to think that there's been some kind of mistake: the tests are wrong, those are someone else's X-rays, this couldn't possibly be happening to you. For many others, as it was for me, the initial response is more one of shock and sad-ness. Today's times do not leave much opportunity for denial. And shock and sadness quickly yield to a resolve to get on with it: to consult the experts, to begin whatever treatments are re-quired, and to do so not with denial but with hope. Norman Cousins witnessed a similar response in some cancer patients who had been given grave prognoses. As he tells it in his book *Head First*, these people didn't reject their doctors' analyses; rather, they "defied the verdict that was supposed to go with it" and didn't give up.

~ ANGER. Not all of us are quick to flare up, either. Since almost half of us will be diagnosed with cancer at some point in our lives, and many will face fears of death, anger makes no sense. Achilles said to Odysseus, "Death comes alike to the idle man and to him that works much," as it comes alike to the mellow man and to him that is on the brittle edge. But anger is not a terribly help-ful or hopeful or healthful response, unless as a momentary flare

that helps to galvanize a person into action. But that's more resolve than anger—a way of saying, "I'm going to beat this."

~ BARGAINING. As for deal making, perhaps that's inevitable
whenever we are caught in a difficult spot. Trying to bargain
with God is a strong thread in many religions, going back at
least to the time of David; it's an "if you save me I will sing your
praises" kind of pleading. As I have already confessed, since I
was little I made a practice of negotiating with the Lord and
with my chosen saints. Real-life bargaining can be a life-
affirming and even lighthearted thing to do. No doubt my doctors were sometimes exhausted by my negotiations with them
over how soon I could get back to work or about scheduling the
next round of treatments so they would not interfere with a
long-planned family vacation.

~ DEPRESSION. Though Kübler-Ross captures well the reactive
depression that inevitably hits when one stares darkly across the
valley of tears, those feelings can be more complicated depending on an individual's underlying temperament. And patients
have a way of rallying fairly quickly from the depths of melan-
choly even in the most difficult of times. Of course, there were
periods when my spirits were down, when my heart felt as heavy
and black as could be. I'd be lying if I said otherwise. I felt those
Dylan Thomas moments of "rage, rage against the dying of the
light" and knew my soul was crying out against something that
seemed so unfair. But despair is not sustainable for the human
soul, either. And with the many options for its treatment, including counseling and medication if it can't be shaken, no one
should be resigned to it.

~ ACCEPTANCE. Years ago, journalist Stewart Alsop wrote a
memoir about his encounter with what the doctors initially believed was a rapidly fatal form of leukemia. Their grim prognosis
turned out to be wrong. Alsop felt as if he'd been granted a reprieve, but not before he'd faced invasive tests, hospital stays,
and great uncertainty about his future. In *Stay of Execution*, pub-

lished in 1973, he describes how he came to terms with the unknown. It was in the early days of his illness, and he'd just spent an interminable night in a hospital bed. He was feeling so low that he'd contemplated suicide, which would have meant abandoning his beloved wife and six children: "I never again had a night as bad as that night, nor, I think, shall I ever again. For a kind of protective mechanism took over, after the first shock of being told of the imminence of death, and I suspect that this is true of most people. Partly, this is a perfectly conscious act of will—a decision to allot to the grim future only its share of your thoughts and no more."

In his battle with cancer, Alsop never lost faith that he would have a reprieve. Indeed, he was granted many reprieves before he gave way. But as a good reporter, he could see his body fade, his energy dwindle, and time grow blurry, leading him to come to terms with death philosophically even when he knew it was not imminent. He wrote that death was, even in anticipation, an interesting experience: "There is a time to live and there is a time to die . . . and there comes a time when it is wrong as well as useless to resist. That time has not yet come for me. But it will. It will for all of us."

For all of us, the common denominator is that death is not optional, and we must recognize it as a phase of living, just like birthing. Indeed, this is the foundation of the hospice movement, whose mission is to provide skilled professionals either at home or in a hospice environment to bring comfort to patients and their families as they accept the inevitable. Focusing on the individual's unique physical, emotional, and spiritual needs, hospice offers a gentle way to say good-bye.

But no one can really prepare for the certain moment, since that moment is still life's mystery. It comes in its own time and way. And for most cancer patients, when it does, death is a gentle fading off, without fear. At that moment, as Alsop put it so elegantly in his abstract musings, "a dying man needs to die, as a sleepy man needs to sleep." I'm sure he knew the brother of Thanatos was Hypnos, the god of sleep.

Search for Meaning

Years ago, long before I had ever faced serious illness myself, I gave a commencement address at my alma mater Vassar College. I told those fresh-faced graduates something that most of us understand intuitively as we add on some years, yet blissfully forget in the bustle of our everyday lives. It was my closing note, speaking as a doctor who over the years had shared the final moments of many of my patients. At that time people aren't preoccupied with how much money they've made or degrees they piled up. Rather, it's those they love and who in turn love them that matter most. That circle of love is as good a measure of a life as I know. Life becomes very simple when you see it in these terms. This is something for all of us to keep in our peripheral vision when we're healthy; it moves front and center when we're sick.

When I was first told I had cancer, I initially assumed I would need to retire. The news about my illness knocked me off balance, and I figured I didn't have a choice. But I realized very quickly that this could be exactly the wrong action to take; even if I had only a limited amount of time left, I wanted to spend it doing what I loved and living as vigorously as I could—which for me meant being with my family and friends and working on the things I loved with the people I cared for. When you're hit with a cancer diagnosis and the ground is getting soft underneath your feet, who and what you love become your anchors. Don't turn away from them, for they are part of your very being.

Steve Jobs, of Apple Computer and Pixar fame, imparted that message poignantly to the 2005 graduating class of Stanford University. He talked about his own cancer diagnosis and brush with death. He called death "the single best invention of life," because it forces us to change and "clears out the old to make way for the new." As is the case for others in this situation, his experience brought home the fact that we are only on this planet for a short period of time and we shouldn't "waste it living someone else's life." A cancer diagnosis can bring your priorities into sharp relief and make you very efficient. Suddenly it's easier to say no to the people you don't really enjoy spending time with; the activities that don't bring you pleasure cease to tug at your conscience, too. Your world may get slightly smaller, but it becomes more meaningful.

In my experience, I found that a few friends sort of fell away, but the ones who stayed close were the ones especially dear to my family and me. There is a liberation that comes with cleansing your calendar of all the things that you used to feel you had to do. It became easy for me to turn down lectures, meetings, travel, and social engagements that were really not very much fun and often exhausting. I learned to conserve my time for what in my heart—with no apologies—mattered most to me, and without the heavy dose of Irish Catholic guilt that used to fall upon me when I had to say no.

In this vein I was especially amused by Jobs' closing remarks at Stanford. He described the *Whole Earth Catalog*, an unusual compilation of images and ideas that was first published in 1968 and found an immediate audience in the counterculture of the day. On the back of the last issue of the catalog, he recalled, was a bucolic image of a country road, along with the line "Stay hungry. Stay foolish." Though Jobs was speaking to a group of young people about to embark on a different type of sojourn, this motto is also apt for those in the midst of a journey through cancer. I would add two more words of advice for the walk along that road: "Be yourself."

And that brings me back to the existential wisdom of Viktor Frankl. His therapeutic technique was based on the premise that the search for meaning in our own personal lives is a primary motivational force if we listen to it. One of the ways we can discover this meaning is in how we handle unavoidable suffering. Suffering is an inextricable part of life. As he puts it, "Without suffering and death human life cannot be complete." But it's the way we deal with this hardship that can enrich our lives and give it deeper meaning. When a situation is dire and there's nothing that can alter it, we need to change our approach in order to "transform a personal tragedy into a triumph, to turn one's predicament into a human achievement." Life is full of difficulties, and only you can choose how you will handle them. That's the journey we all have to go through, cancer patient or not.

I'm often asked how my experience with this disease has transformed me. I say, "I'm still me." Just because I've been ill doesn't change who I am. I remember when I went to a high school reunion once. At the end of the day, I asked my friend Susan Schulman, now a publicist in New York, who organized the event, whether she thought our former classmates had changed. Her response was prompt: nobody was that different. "They were just more of how they used to be. The snooty ones were snootier, the sweet ones even more so." Some say that with age you do become more of who you are, and an illness can do this to you, too. The mask comes off, and your true self is laid bare. Yet as Frankl implies, we're always reaching beyond our limits. A young man may realize that he's not the smartest kid in the class, for example, but he makes up for it by studying hard and learning how to compensate in other ways for his academic deficiencies; a woman may not be the prettiest, but she has learned how her inner beauty shines through when she is at her best, perhaps aided by a nice shade of lipstick. But always with authenticity. An illness such as cancer can set us up to think about our own capacity to enhance our strengths and make our days meaningful to ourselves and to those we care most about. This process is in essence a spiritual experience.

Frankl's words came back to me as I sat with a dear friend of mine who was near death. Al Lerner was almost seventy and had been suffering with a rapidly progressing cancer over a period of eighteen months. He had endured heavy treatments and more recently some harsh experimental therapies that failed to work. He knew the end was very close. I dropped by to see him one sunny afternoon. His wife, Norma, also a dear friend of many years, was in the kitchen making some lunch, so for about twenty minutes he and I sat alone in the garden. We talked quietly in a way that only close friends do when they have faced similar times and felt the same flashes of un-spoken desolation as they are forced to confront their own mortal-ity. Al couldn't quite wrap his head around the fact that his body was failing him. Here he was, sitting in the sunshine, among the care-fully tended flowers and shrubs that were just starting to think about what September meant to their blossoms and leaves, with similar thoughts that he, too, would fade away in this same season.

Yet his spirit and presence were still so mighty, as they had been for all his life. He was an extraordinary man of great public success and prominence, but of even greater personal depth and humanity. Though he was a man of vast and often hidden tenderness, he didn't do spirituality. But spirituality tumbled out of his heart just then. "Bernie, how can it be that I am here now, yet my body might not be? How can it be that what I am inside can disappear?" It has to go on to be somewhere, he said with the wonder of a philosopher prob-ing the secrets of life. I knew he was right; he would live on. Just be-cause we mortals are limited by five senses, three physical dimensions, and one dimension of time does not mean that other di-mensions of time and being can't be known to us. I told him I knew fervently that he would endure powerfully. Whether these thoughts brought him comfort, I will never know for sure. But, perhaps self-ishly, they helped me face his loss several weeks later.

For many other people, faith is front and center for most of their lives, and they are used to looking to a higher being for a sense of purpose and peace. For them, reading the Bible or other religious writings, praying, and having others pray for them can be calming. But sometimes they, too, struggle, perhaps with a sense of betrayal. How can this God whom they have worshiped abandon them? But these thoughts are checked as their faith brings them insight and re-newed strength.

I guess I fall somewhere in the middle on this spiritual spectrum. I found solace in the immutable wisdom of the ancient texts, reading the Bible, or meditating on the psalms from my little red Catholic psalm book that Mom had saved for all those years. Sometimes, when I was alone, I read them out loud. I prayed, too, as I had in the past, and often just sat quietly and anonymously in the back of a church or chapel that I happened by. But I also wear Michele's cross, and a pretty blue good-luck charm from my close friend Seyhan. I cherished a connection with the ever-changing river that ran outside our window in Washington, and the predictably changing oak and hickory trees that have lived so long around our home in Cleveland. Timeless hymns had special meaning to me—from the Ave Maria that was my father's favorite to the piercing melody of the Kol Nidre, which I learned from a Hunter College High School friend, Lynn Visson.

Through the ages, people everywhere have looked to the arts—a sublime piece of music, a timeless painting, a classic work of literature—for inspiration, guidance, balm for their ailing spirit. Sometimes you just need a lovely diversion to take your mind off the blood counts and treatment schedules, allow you to think deeply and soothingly for a while, and to remember that life goes on. I recall a serene moment early in my cancer journey. My outlook was uncertain, and my mood reflected it: I had been feeling vulnerable and weak, both physically and emotionally. On that particular day I had a platelet transfusion. During the process I absorbed myself in my book, *Memoirs of a Geisha*, which had blessedly transported me to another world. I was so sorry to turn the last page of this gorgeously written novel. As I read and reread its last few lines, a surprising euphoria came over me. I felt calm and ready for whatever the future might bring as I contemplated the imagery that jumped off the last page of the book: "But now I know that our world is no more permanent than a wave rising on the ocean. Whatever our struggles and triumphs, however we may suffer them, all too soon they bleed into a wash, just like watery ink on paper."

Call it religion, call it spirituality, call it grace. We are all beings in one point in time. We are all ripples in the ocean. And thinking about that brought me a calm and equanimity that tapped into the core of my soul. The same sense of calm washes over me almost every time I read the wisdom of the psalmists written thousands of years ago, echoing the same message in a different way. I came to better terms with my misbehaving clump of cells that day, and the effect has been enduring.

If or when my beast acts up again, I will know what to expect. I will not see whatever treatment is there for me as salvage, but as round two or round three. And if I get knocked out in that round, I will have tried the best I could, with the firm belief that someday my girls and my sweet husband will look back and say, "You know, we could have cured Mom had she lived today." I hope so. I've already seen the glimmer that such a time is coming—the time when cancer has no riddles, presents few uncertainties, and brings no fear.

RESOURCES

General Cancer Information

Patients and their families as well as the doctors who care for them can now turn to the Web for reliable information on virtually any aspect of cancer medicine. I have listed some of these resources, which offer access to both the very latest technical scientific research as well as to patient-friendly translations of what is important. I have included only nonprofit sources, and advise that you familiarize yourself with the sites I've asterisked (*) as a starter. The numerous scientific studies I have referred to in the book can be found in abstract form by topic on www.pubmed.gov. Remember that the information provided here and throughout the book is not a substitute for the advice and care of your personal physician.

American Cancer Society*: toll free (800) 227-2345; www.cancer.org. This easy-to-navigate Web site is bursting with valuable information, guidance, and support that will be helpful to patients, their loved ones, survivors, and medical professionals. And there is an opportunity to donate to the cause and volunteer as well.

American Society of Clinical Oncology*: (ASCO) (703) 299-0150; www.asco.org. ASCO is a leading worldwide professional organization comprising the full spectrum of cancer practitioners, researchers, and educators devoted to improving cancer care and prevention and advocating policies that ensure individual access to high-quality cancer care and to clinical cancer research. Through its many publications and its Web site it is a valuable source of information. ASCO shares a patient information site named **People Living with Cancer**: toll free (888) 651-3038; direct (703) 519-2927; www.plwc.org.

National Cancer Institute*: National Institutes of Health, Department of Health and Human Services: toll free (800) 422-6237; www.cancer.gov. With one click this federal government site offers a wealth of material on treatment options, clinical trials, prevention, genetics, causes of particular types of cancer, screening and testing, research and related information, and statistics. Cancer.gov will also indicate which medical facilities have the most experience in dealing with a particular type of cancer. NCI sponsors a cancer information service for patients at cis.nci.nih.gov.

National Library of Medicine*: National Institutes of Health: toll free (888) 346-3656; direct and international (301) 594-5983; www.nlm.nih.gov. NLM is the largest medical library in the world and has pioneered online medical information for medical professionals and for the public. *PubMed* provides science abstracts of the latest research worldwide at www.pubmed.gov. This site can provide you with literature regarding your specific disease. You can type in "breast cancer," for example, and see abstracts for all of the relevant peer-reviewed journal articles. While some of this information is rather technical, it will give you a good idea of the kind of research that is going on, who is doing it and at which institutions. *Medline* is another National Library of Medicine offering, with a special patient-oriented site, *MedlinePlus:* www.nlm.nih.gov/medlineplus. MedlinePlus hosts a medical encyclopedia with user-friendly information on more than 700 conditions, including specific cancers, a medical dictionary, information on drugs and supplements, and directories of medical professionals. For *clinical trials*, see the National Library of Medicine's site, www.clinicaltrials.gov, which in a click will inform you and your doctor of clinical trials that might be of interest, and provide names and contact information so you can reach the institutions directly.

National Human Genome Research Institute*: National Institutes of Health: direct and international (301) 402-0911; www.genome .gov. This site provides information on the Human Genome Project, The Cancer Genome Atlas, and the Genome Research Institute's many cancer-related collaborations with the NCI.

National Center for Complementary and Alternative Medicine*: National Institutes of Health: toll free (888) 644-6226; direct and international (301) 519-3153; nccam.nih.gov. Additional information on complementary medicine can be found at "CAM on PubMed," http://nccam .nih.gov/camonpubmed, and from the National Cancer Institute, www.cancer.gov/cam.

National Institute of Environmental Health Sciences*: National Institutes of Health: direct and international (919) 541-3345; www.niehs.nih.gov. NIEHS devotes much of its efforts to studying the interaction between the environment and the development of cancer, and its site contains information on basic and applied research in this field. The NIEHS houses the **National Toxicology Program**, an interagency effort including the National Institutes of Health, the Centers for Disease Control and Prevention, and the Environmental Protection Agency, and regularly assesses the effect of environmental factors on human health. NTP produces a biennial *Report on Carcinogens* that can be accessed at http://ntp.niehs.nih.gov.

Centers for Disease Control and Prevention*: Department of Health and Human Services: toll free (800) 311-3435; direct and international (404) 639-3534; www.cdc.gov. This site offers a plethora of information about cancer and cancer survivors, some of it from a public health perspective. Here you'll also find instructions on how to calculate your body mass index: www.cdc.gov/nccdphp/dnpa/bmi/calc-bmi.htm, and information and trends on the health of the U.S. population developed by the National Center for Health Statistics, www.cdc.gov/nchs.

International Union Against Cancer (UICC): +41 22 809 1811; www.uicc.org. Headquartered in Geneva, Switzerland, the UICC focuses on scientific and medical knowledge related to global cancer control for both professionals and the public. It works closely with the NCI.

American Institute for Cancer Research: toll free (800) 843-8114, direct and international (202) 328-7744; www.aicr.org. AICR advocates research on diet and nutrition, and offers consumers personalized information.

Association of Cancer Online Resources: direct (212) 226-5525; www.acor.org. ACOR's Web site helps those with cancer contact others with similar diagnoses to create online health communities.

Cancer*Care***:** toll free (800) 813-4673; direct and international (212) 302-2400; www.cancercare.org. This organization provides general cancer information, online chat rooms, and scheduled telephone education sessions on cancer care and available social services, including financial assistance and practical help.

Cancer 411.org: www.cancer411.org. This organization was founded in memory of two patients, Rory Leifer and Joyce Kramer, to provide information on treatment options and available clinical cancer trials.

Coalition of National Cancer Cooperative Groups: toll free (877) 520-4457; www.cancertrialshelp.org. The coalition consists of a network of leading cancer clinical trial specialists, and offers to patients and their doctors information about ongoing clinical trials for a particular tumor. The group also advocates for participation in clinical trials. The site contains a link to the CancerQuilt, where individuals tell their own personal cancer stories, forming a virtual cancer quilt.

Lance Armstrong Foundation: direct and international (512) 236-8820; toll free for Livestrong Survivor Care hotline (866) 235-7205; www.livestrong.org. Founded by Lance Armstrong with the help of his mother to serve patients and survivors, family and loved ones, who have been touched by cancer of any kind. The goal is to provide inspiration, advocacy, and information, and to raise funds for cancer research.

National Coalition for Cancer Survivorship: direct (301) 650-9127; www.canceradvocacy.org. This advocacy group focuses on survivors of all types of cancer and their families.

Cancer Research and Prevention Foundation: toll free (800) 227-2732; direct (703) 519-2103; www.preventcancer.org. Established in 1985, this foundation is dedicated to research and education on the prevention and early detection of cancer.

Friends of Cancer Research: direct (703) 302-1503; www.focr.org. The program focuses on public policy advocacy for cancer research, and for offering patients accessible prevention and treatment options. The group collaborates with the motion picture industry and the media to educate the public about cancer and to raise funds for cancer programs.

Gilda's Club Worldwide: toll free (888) 445-3248; www.gildasclub .org. Founded on behalf of the beloved actress Gilda Radner who died of ovarian cancer, the organization offers support to those who have been touched by cancer, through a series of support groups, lectures, and social gatherings.

R. A. Bloch Cancer Foundation: toll free (800) 433-0464; www.blochcancer.org. This organization provides a toll-free hotline to connect patients who have experienced similar tumors and can offer information and support, and identifies links to other cancer Web sites.

CancerGuide: www.cancerguide.org. This is a Web-based resource founded by the late Steve Dunn to respond to questions about all kinds of cancer, including those that are less common. Trained volunteers maintain the Web site.

U.S. News Best Health: www.usnews.com/usnews/health/hehome .htm. A Web site from *U.S. News & World Report* that offers an annual ranking of the top cancer centers, a cancer condition center, features and news briefs about cancer useful to patients and their families.

Tumor-Specific Information and Advocacy Groups

Although it's important that you work with your own team of doctors and specialists, the following organizations may provide you with some additional useful information on your own tumor, a vehicle for support, and in some cases a place to get involved with helping others. I cannot vouch for the information on every site, but I am impressed by the wide range of reliable resources that are available at a click and in the privacy of your home.

Breast Cancer
- **BreastCancer.Net**: www.breastcancer.net. This is an online clearinghouse for breast cancer news and information.
- **Susan G. Komen Breast Cancer Foundation**: toll free (800) 462-9273; www.komen.org. Founded by Nancy Brinker in memory of her sister, Susan, this foundation supports research and community-based outreach programs through a network of U.S. and international affiliates. It has raised millions of dollars for research through its sponsorship of the Komen Race for the Cure in cities nationwide.

- **National Breast Cancer Coalition**: toll free (800) 622-2838; direct (202) 296-7477; www.natlbcc.org or www.stopbreast-cancer.org. The coalition is a grassroots national advocacy group that has been effective in influencing public policy and support for breast cancer research.
- **Living Beyond Breast Cancer**: toll free (888) 753-5222; www.lbbc.org. An educational resource for women surviving breast cancer.
- **Sisters Network**: toll free (866) 781-1808; direct (713) 781-0255; www.sistersnetworkinc.org. A national organization that focuses on the needs of African American women who have survived breast cancer. It has chapters across the country.
- **Y-Me National Breast Cancer Organization**: toll free 24-hour hotline (800) 221-2141 in English and (800) 986-9504 in Spanish; www.y-me.org. This group provides information and services, including a wig and breast prostheses bank free of charge for women with limited resources.
- **Young Survival Coalition**: (646) 257-3000; www.youngsur-vival.org. YSC is a group of survivors and supporters that focuses specifically on the needs of young women.
- **FORCE: Facing Our Risk of Cancer Empowered**: toll free (866) 824-7475; www.facingourrisk.org. FORCE is dedicated to women with hereditary breast and ovarian cancer, and those with known risk for these cancers.

Cervical Cancer

- **Gynecologic Cancer Foundation**: toll free (800) 444-4441; direct (312) 578-1439; www.thegcf.org; www.cervicalcancer campaign .org. The foundation was organized with the Society of Gyne-cologic Oncologists to increase public awareness of these cancers of women, including their prevention, treatment, and research.
- **National Cervical Cancer Coalition**: toll free (800) 685-5531; www.nccc-online.org. NCCC is a grassroots effort focusing on women with cervical cancer or HPV disease.

Childhood Cancer

- **Candlelighters Childhood Cancer Foundation:** toll free (800) 366-2223; international and direct (301) 962-3520; www.candle-lighters.org. Established in 1970, Candlelighters is an education and advocacy group for all children and adolescents with cancer.

- **The Children's Cause for Cancer Advocacy:** (301) 562-2765; www.childrenscause.org. CCA advocates for research funding for drug discovery and development for children with all forms of cancer.

- **CureSearch of the Children's Oncology Group and the National Childhood Cancer Foundation:** toll free (800) 458-6223; www.childrensoncologygroup.org; www.curesearch.org. This group helps families find hospitals and clinical research programs suitable for their children's tumors.

- **National Children's Cancer Society:** toll free (800) 532-6459; direct (314) 241-1600; www.nationalchildrenscancersociety .org. The society promotes quality of life for children with cancer through financial and in-kind assistance, advocacy, and education. The society has a separate effort, **Beyond the Cure**, (800) 532-6459; www.beyondthecure.org, which focuses on the needs of childhood cancer survivors long term.

- **Outlook: Life Beyond Childhood Cancer:** www.outlook-life.org. An online resource that provides information on school, camps, and jobs, and addresses long-term health concerns of survivors of childhood cancer.

- **Starlight Starbright Children's Foundation:** toll free (800) 315-2580; direct and international (310) 479-1212; www.slsb.org. This international foundation focuses on the immediate needs of children from the time of their diagnosis through hospitalization and treatment. The group sponsors playrooms, teen lounges, books and toys, and escape opportunities at times when children and their families need them the most.

Central Nervous System and Brain Cancers

- **American Brain Tumor Association:** toll free (800) 886-2282; www.abta.org. ABTA provides patient information about brain tumors and their treatment, as well as links to information about medical care, clinical trials, and a wide range of support services.
- **Accelerate Brain Cancer Cure** (ABC^2): direct (202) 419-3140; www.abc2.org. Founded by Dan Case (who suffered and died from glioblastoma multiforme) together with his brother, Internet entrepreneur Steve Case, the organization is dedicated to accelerating a cure for this "complex, virulent, and orphaned" disease by bringing a results-driven business model to identifying and supporting cutting-edge research, as well as promoting research and development partnerships focused on treatment and cure.
- **The Brain Tumor Society:** toll free (800) 770-8287; www.tbts .org. Provides information about treatment and support services for patients, hosts educational meetings, and raises money for research grants.
- **National Brain Tumor Foundation:** toll free (800) 934-2873; direct (510) 839-9777; www.braintumor.org. This organization offers educational support, online information, brochures, and other educational support services to patients and their families, and also raises funds for research.
- **The Brain Tumor Foundation:** (212) 265-2401; www.braintumorfoundation.org. This foundation fosters education for the public and medical professionals about brain tumors, sponsors local support groups, and promotes consideration of early detection of brain tumors in high-risk people using MRI imaging technology.
- **Children's Neuroblastoma Cancer Foundation:** toll free (866) 671-2623; www.cncf-childcancer.org. A network of families and medical professionals supporting needs of children with this tumor.

- **The Childhood Brain Tumor Foundation:** toll free (877) 217-4166; direct (301) 515-2900; www.childhoodbraintumor.org. Founded by families and friends of children with brain tumors to raise money for research.
- **Children's Brain Tumor Foundation:** toll free (866) 228-4673; www.cbtf.org. This group is dedicated to improving treatment and quality of life for children with brain and central nervous system cancers through research and education.
- **Pediatric Brain Tumor Foundation of the United States:** toll free (800) 253-6530; direct (828) 665-6891; www.pbtfus.org. PBTFUS provides grants for basic research, sponsors family linking for those with cancer, and holds a fund-raising effort among motorcyclists, called the "Ride for Kids."

Colorectal Cancer
- **Colon Cancer Alliance:** toll free (877) 422-2030; direct (212) 627-7451; www.ccalliance.org. The alliance provides education, information, resources, and support to those with this cancer.
- **Colorectal Cancer Network:** (301) 879-1500; www.colorectalcancer.net. The network offers support groups, listservs, and chat rooms to connect people who have colon cancer.
- **Hereditary Colon Cancer Association:** toll free (800) 264-6783; www.hereditarycc.org. This association is dedicated to patients with all forms of hereditary colon cancer and those at risk for it, promoting awareness, education, and research.
- **The United Ostomy Associations of America:** toll free (800) 826-0826; www.uoaa.org. UOAA offers information, education, resources, and support for those with colostomies after cancer surgery.

Esophageal Cancer
- **Cathy's EC Café:** www.eccafe.org. Web site provides information and support to those at risk for, and with, this cancer.

• **Esophageal Cancer Awareness Association**: toll free (866) 370-3222; direct (607) 257-1141; www.ecaware.org. This site offers information on the disease and its treatment.

Head and Neck Cancer

• **Support for People with Oral, Head, and Neck Cancers**: toll free (800) 377-0928; www.spohnc.org. SPOHNC is a patient-directed self-help organization that deals with the emotional and physical needs of those with head and neck cancers.
• **The Oral Cancer Foundation**: (949) 646-8000; www.oralcancerfoundation.org. This group was founded to provide patient information, support, and advocacy.

Kidney Cancer

• **Kidney Cancer Association**: toll free (800) 850-9132; direct (847) 332-1051; in Canada (416) 848-9625; in Europe +44 020 8123 3895; www.nkca.org. The association provides an online and telephone resource for kidney cancer patients and their families. Its site also includes a medical professional site both for education and to search for available clinical trials.
• **Action to Cure Kidney Cancer**: (212) 799-4354; www.ackc.org. The organization's mission is to raise awareness of kidney cancer and advocate for increased public and private funding of research.

Leukemia and Lymphoma

• **Leukemia Research Foundation**: direct (847) 424-0600; www.leukemia-research.org. The foundation funds research into causes and cures of leukemia, lymphoma, and myelodysplastic syndromes.
• **The Leukemia & Lymphoma Society**: toll free (800) 955-4572; www.leukemia-lymphoma.org. This organization funds blood cancer research, education, and patient services.
• **Lymphoma Research Foundation**: toll free (800) 500-9976; www.lymphoma.org. This organization funds lymphoma research,

and has both patient and professional education information on its site.

- **Lymphoma Foundation of America**: toll free hotline (800) 385-1060; direct (734) 222-1100; www.lymphomahelp.org. This foundation provides support groups and services to lymphoma patients and their families.
- **The Myelodysplastic Syndromes Foundation**: toll free (800) 637-0839; direct and international (609) 298-6746; www.mds-foundation.org. This international foundation focuses on prevention, treatment, and study of this less well-known group of blood cancers.

Multiple Myeloma

- **International Myeloma Foundation**: toll free (800) 452-2873; direct and international (818) 487-7455; www.myeloma.org. The foundation offers information to the public and medical professionals on the latest in the treatment of the disease, new drugs in development, and lists ongoing clinical trials.
- **Multiple Myeloma Research Foundation**: (203) 229-0464; www.multiplemyeloma.org. This foundation raises money for research and provides information on new treatment developments.

Liver Cancer

- **LiverTumor.org**: www.livertumor.org. An online resource that provides patients with information on the disease, its treatment, and accessing physicians who specialize in liver cancer.

Lung Cancer

- **Lung Cancer Alliance**: toll free (800) 298-2436; direct (202) 463-2080; www.lungcanceralliance.org. LCA is dedicated to patient support and advocacy for those with lung cancer and those who are at risk, addressing directly the stigma associated with the disease that they fear depresses public support and research funding. Its Web site offers the latest information on clinical trials and new treatment options, and champions early disease detection as well as anti-smoking campaigns.

- **American Lung Association**: toll free (800) 586-4872; www.lungusa.org. As part of its broad mission the association promotes education and research study of lung cancer, and is a useful resource for patients and families.
- **It's Time to Focus on Lung Cancer**: toll free (877) 646-5864; www.lungcancer.org is a service of Cancer*Care* that provides free professional counseling, education, financial help, and other assistance to those with this disease.
- **Lung Cancer Online Foundation**: www.lungcanceronline .org. LCOF provides online information on lung cancer for patients and their families.

Ovarian Cancer

- **National Ovarian Cancer Coalition**: toll free (888) 682-7426; direct (561) 393-0005; www.ovarian.org. NOCC raises awareness and promotes education about ovarian cancer.
- **Ovarian Cancer National Alliance**: direct (202) 331-1332; www.ovariancancer.org. This is an alliance of several ovarian cancer groups to promote education, public awareness, and research.
- **Ovarian Cancer Research Fund**: toll free (800) 873-9569; www.ocrf.org. This fund supports research programs and fosters awareness of ovarian cancer.
- **Gynecologic Cancer Foundation**: toll free (800) 444-4441; www.thegcf.org. Promotes public awareness of prevention, treatment, and research on gynecologic tumors, including ovary. It sponsors the patient information Web site **Women's Cancer Network**, www.wcn.org.

Pancreatic Cancer

- **Pancreatic Cancer Action Network**: toll free (877) 272-6226; direct (310) 752-0025; www.pancan.org. A voluntary health organization dedicated to patient education, advocacy, and research on this disease.

- **Hirshberg Foundation for Pancreatic Cancer Research**: direct (310) 472-6310; www.pancreatic.org. This organization is dedicated to advancing pancreatic cancer research, and to providing informational resources to those with the disease.
- **Lustgarten Foundation for Pancreatic Cancer Research**: toll free (866) 789-1000; direct (516) 803-2304; www.lustgarten-foundation.org. The foundation offers patient information and has an active grant program to fund pancreatic cancer research.
- **Pancreatica.org**: direct (831) 658-0600; www.pancreatica .org. A worldwide online resource for the latest developments in pancreatic cancer, particularly new treatment options.

Prostate Cancer

- **American Foundation for Urologic Disease**: toll free (800) 828-7866; (866) 746-4282; www.auafoundation.org. This organization raises money for prostate cancer research and provides information on the disease. The AFUD also hosts a patient education site at www.urologyhealth.org, which also offers information on prostate cancer specialists. Both are linked to the American Urological Association.
- **National Prostate Cancer Coalition**: toll free (888) 245-9455; direct (202) 245-9455; www.fightprostatecancer.org. The coalition offers awareness and advocacy for the disease, and outreach to patients and their families.
- **Prostate Cancer Education Council**: toll free (866) 477-6788; direct (303) 316-4685; www.pcaw.com. The council raises awareness of the disease and the need for routine early detection screening, and offers the public general information on prostate cancer.
- **Prostate Cancer Foundation**: toll free (800) 757-2873; www.prostatecancerfoundation.org. This foundation focuses

on research to improve treatment options and to find a cure for recurrent disease.

- **Prostate Health Education Network**: direct (781) 487-2239; www.prostatehealthed.org. PHEN's goal is to make African American men, the group most susceptible to prostate cancer, aware of the disease and the need for early detection and treatment.
- **The Prostate Net**: toll free (888) 477-6763; www.prostate-online.org. This group focuses on the needs of minority men to become aware of prostate cancer and seek early detection screening.
- **Us TOO International**: toll free (800) 808-7866; direct (630) 795-1002; www.ustoo.org. Us TOO is funded by prostate cancer survivors to serve other survivors and their families.

Rare Cancers

- **National Organization for Rare Disorders**: toll free, voice mail only (800) 999-6673; direct (203) 744-0100; www.rare-diseases.org. NORD maintains an online index and database of rare diseases, including cancers.
- **Rare Cancer Alliance**: toll free (800) 345-6324; www.rare-cancer.org. This Web site provides information about rare forms of adult and pediatric cancers.

Sarcoma

- **Sarcoma Alliance**: direct (415) 381-7236; www.sarcoma-alliance.org. Provides guidance, education, and support to patients and families.
- **Sarcoma Foundation of America**: direct (301) 253-8687; www.curesarcoma.org. This foundation advocates greater public awareness of the family of these diseases, and the need for increased research funding and alliance between university researchers and industry to foster new and better treatments.

- **Bone Cancer FAQ**: www.cancerindex.org/ccw/faq. An educational Web site for patients with sarcoma of bone or cartilage.

Skin Cancer
- **American Melanoma Foundation**: direct (619) 448-0991; www.melanomafoundation.org. The foundation provides information about prevention, early diagnosis, and treatment, as well as the latest in research findings.
- **Melanoma Research Foundation**: toll free (800) 673-1290; www.melanoma.org. The organization supports research, offers information about the prevention and treatment of the disease, and advocates on behalf of those affected by melanoma.
- **The Skin Cancer Foundation**: toll free (800) 754-6490; www.skincancer.org. Its goal is to increase global awareness about prevention, early detection, and treatment of all forms of skin cancer.

Testicular Cancer
- **Testicular Cancer Resource Center**: www.tcrc.acor.org. The Web site offers information about the illness, describes treatment options, and provides useful links to other medical sites.

Thyroid Cancer
- **Thyroid Cancer Survivors' Association**: toll free (877) 588-7904; www.thyca.org. This information and patient support group also focuses on the need for research funding for the disease, which is increasing in the population.

ACKNOWLEDGMENTS

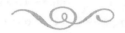

Acknowledgment should be the easiest part of writing a book, yet it may be the hardest as it is the moment to recognize the many forces that went into a book's creation. In fact, they are too vast to be recounted and are sometimes too subtle to be defined. Allow me to try, and forgive the inevitable omissions.

The motivation for this book came from those who have been touched by cancer, directly or through a loved one. They are the ones who have driven medical research, insisted on better care, and made it possible for the cancer journey to be eased for the next wave of patients. To those who carry that torch forward, and to my many colleagues in medicine on the frontlines of the cancer war, I am deeply grateful.

This was not a book I ever planned to write; I worked hard at putting my own illness behind me. But it has been my time at *U.S. News & World Report* that gave me the confidence to embark on the effort, stimulated by a piece I reluctantly wrote, in response to an editor's gentle prodding, to accompany a cover story on cancer survivors. "I'm Still Here" was the result, and it became the germ of this book.

Being part of the *U.S. News* family has been one of the most satisfying stages of my life in medicine. Immersed in a land of ideas, smart people, and breaking news, it's an adventure to be part of the magazine. This challenging, high performance place has pushed me to hone my writing skills. It brings me back to medicine full time as I imagine every reader as my patient, and try to speak to him or to her in measured but frank words about the health and medicine that each must own. With the magazine's permission, I have adapted the thoughts and words in some of my columns for use in this book.

For all of this I give many thanks to editor-in-chief Mortimer Zuckerman, who has long been dedicated to medicine and medical communication and invited me to join his team back in 2002; and to the magazine's editor Brian Duffy, who welcomed me with his quiet and steady support, and continues to influence my work with his sharp journalist eye. Margi Mannix, managing editor for health and medicine, is a thrill to work with—energetic, creative, witty and always available, however long the day may be. Margi has the heart of a doctor, ever sensitive to the needs of the reader-patient, and kindly read through an early draft of the book. I've also been lucky to have an office next to Avery Comarow, a gifted medical writer and editor who is as enchanted by medicine as any doctor I know. His encouraging words slipped into our casual corridor kibitzing, and that was after he read an early chapter. To them and to my many other friends at *U.S. News*, I offer my appreciation and respect.

During the course of writing this book I've spoken to countless physicians and researchers, read volumes of medical reports from leading medical institutions whose work is heavily supported by the National Institutes of Health, and tapped into the vast resources of the National Library of Medicine, which were developed over the years with the leadership of its director, Donald A. B. Lindberg. I value the generosity of my colleagues and the greatness of these institutions that serve us all.

It's fair to say that without the Cleveland Clinic, the Taussig Cancer Center, and my brain trust, this book would not have been possible. Dr. Patrick Sweeney has been my ever-so-intellectual guardian angel; Gene Barnett's skill and quiet strength have helped me through many stressful times; and David Peereboom, smart and kind and deeply spiritual, has offered creative insight at just the right moments. Bruce Cohen, renowned for his compassion and knowledge, brought exquisite judgment to a field filled with enigmas, and Brian Bolwell, my marrow keeper, is a superb oncologist comfortable with questioning established dogma in the interest of his patients. Maureen Bell, Mary Miller, Michele Gavin, Edward Palmer, Frederick Van Lente, Ronald Bukowski, Paul Ruggieri, Hans Luders, Walter Maurer, Zeyd Ebrahim, Gregory Zuccaro, Joseph Crowe, Nagy Mekhail, Joanne Hilden, and Derek Raghavan are a wonderful sampling of the many devoted professionals who are the backbone of an institution whose mission first and foremost is better care of the patient.

It is also a certain truth that writing a book, or getting through an illness, is a lot easier with the encouragement of dear friends. I thank them, including Seyhan Soylu, Kate Berry, Helen and Roger Mee, Victor Fazio, Jane Pfeiffer, Al and Norma Lerner, Mal and Barb Mixon, Vera and Walter Rausnitz, Robert and Darlene Duvin, F. George Estafanous, Rick Kaplan, Chet Cooper, Ayhan Sahenk and his family, Pamela and Arnold Sheiffer, Kathy Vaughn, Christine Kassuba, Valerie Stump, Brenda Hammond, Sara Strong, Grayce Sills, Clara Bloomfield, Larry Copeland and Brad Stokes. Of particular note were my two best buddies: Nonie, my husband's mom, who even in her late nineties was my loyal and trusted confidant; and Michele, my sister. I'm hoping they select this book for the book club I'm quite sure they've started up in heaven.

I already miss my Tuesdays with Mindy. I discovered Mindy Werner when she was at Viking editing my first book, *A New Prescription for Women's Health*. Now working independently while overseeing her brood, I was able to enlist her as my personal editor. Our every-Tuesday calls kept me on task, even when I was overwhelmed with other deadlines. Faithfully we spoke, mostly about concepts, structure, and pretty writing. Mindy reviewed and critiqued every chapter many times over, and always was willing to look again, question again. I have also benefited from the talents of

Jane Isay, who helped me think through the original book proposal, and of two former colleagues from *U.S. News*, science writer Tom Hayden and medical editor Wray Herbert, who reviewed and critiqued selected chapters. I am most grateful to Francis Collins, Marcia Angell, Donna Shalala, Jerome Groopman, and Cokie Roberts for taking the time to read the final manuscript.

Gail Ross was my agent for my first book and has been a good friend ever since. She insisted I do this book, and with Gail's determination, I really had no other choice. To her I give particular thanks. At Bantam Books, I was fortunate to find a publisher, Irwyn Applebaum, a publicity director, Barb Burg, and an editor, Toni Burbank, who believed in this book, even though conventional wisdom has it that cancer books don't sell. Thanks, too, to Julie Will, Kelly Chian, and copy editor Sue Warga, for their attentiveness and support.

My parents, Michael and Violet Healy, have been a constant force behind all my academic pursuits, and though he succumbed to cancer 27 years ago, my dad's many words of wisdom echoed in my head and my heart as I worked on this book. Only the deeply rooted work ethic which they imparted could keep me writing in the early morning hours, on weekends, on vacations, and even during a special wedding anniversary cruise. I am blessed to have a family that has passion for books and ideas, and they never *really* minded. All said, I have no greater inspiration, no greater blessing, than Bartlett, Marie, and their dad, Fred Loop. They are my haven and my living time.

INDEX

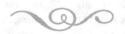

ABOUT THE AUTHOR

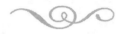

Bernadine Healy, M.D., a leader in patient care, research, and education, has been a medical columnist for *U.S. News & World Report* since
2002, and serves as health editor for the magazine. A Harvard- and
Hopkins-trained physician, Healy is former president of the
American Red Cross, and is a past director of the National Institutes
of Health, where she started the Women's Health Initiative. She was
dean of the College of Medicine and Public Health at Ohio State
University, and chairman of the Research Institute of the Cleveland
Clinic Foundation. On leave from her professorship at Johns
Hopkins in 1984, Dr. Healy served as deputy science advisor to
President Reagan, and since has been a member of the Council of
Advisors on Science and Technology for three Presidents. She has
also served as president of the American Heart Association, and was
awarded the American Heart Association's highest award for service,
the Golden Heart. She has received numerous other awards includ-
ing the Dana Foundation's Distinguished Achievement Award for her
work on promoting research on the health problems of women. Dr.
Healy has been a member of the Institute of Medicine since 1987.
She is married to Dr. Floyd Loop and lives in Cleveland and
Washington, D.C.